THE PSYCHOLOGICAL DIETER

It's Not All About the Calories

Gregory J. Privitera, Ph.D.

University Press of America,® Inc.

Lanham · Boulder · New York · Toronto · Plymouth, UK

Copyright © 2008 by
University Press of America®, Inc.
4501 Forbes Boulevard
Suite 200
Lanham, Maryland 20706
UPA Acquisitions Department (301) 459-3366

Estover Road
Plymouth PL6 7PY
United Kingdom

Library of Congress Control Number: 2007940295
ISBN-13: 978-0-7618-3966-8 (paperback : alk. paper)
ISBN-10: 0-7618-3966-6 (paperback : alk. paper)

⊖™ The paper used in this publication meets the minimum
requirements of American National Standard for Information
Sciences—Permanence of Paper for Printed Library Materials,
ANSI Z39.48—1984

Dedication

To the health of my children,

Aiden and Grace

Contents

Preface

Most diets fail in the long term. Indeed, if any one diet were widely successful, there would be no need for most of the thousands of diets being marketed today. Intervention strategies for promoting long-term weight loss have had less than ringing success over the last twenty years. In an effort to improve long-term success in weight loss, researchers and clinicians have suggested multiple involved solutions, many of which require many hours of exhausting work with expert support. Researchers suggest the need for improved patient retention, long-term assessment of caloric intake and use, identification of obesity phenotypes, implementation of dieting strategies in adolescence, promotion of physical activity, and social support, in addition to pharmacological and various behavioral methods.[1] One common drawback with these strategies is that in many cases they require professional support and a lot of time and effort from the dieter—a dieter who usually has many other uses for his or her time such as working, being a parent, paying bills, and the like.

Until recently, psychologists studied eating by focusing on hunger and fullness (also referred to as satiety). Yet we eat not only because we are hungry, but also because food tastes good. From birth, we tend to eat what we like. We will always eat what we like, eventually. Unfortunately, in the realm of foods and flavors, what we like is not always healthy, and what is healthy is not always what we like. Fortunately, there have been significant advances in many fields of psychology that study eating behavior. These advances help us to understand why foods fill us up (calories are not the primary reason) and how we can learn to like (even prefer) healthier food options in our regular diet. In all, these recent advances demonstrate practical solutions for improving the health of our diets that do not require expensive, long-term, involved medical interventions. Unfortunately, this research is well understood by only a few scientists (mostly researchers). This may be one reason why psychological strategies for improving diet have been largely overlooked in the popular dieting market, in favor of counting calories and similar strategies.

In our food rich society, *pleasure* is the motivation for much of our eating. Indeed, diets fail in the long term because we prefer foods not allowed by those diets. Eventually you will eat what you like, despite your best intentions. In other words, what makes food pleasurable is also what makes us eat it, even when we don't set out to do so. An explosion of research in the last twenty years has demonstrated that experience has profound effects on food likes and dislikes. More important, these likes and dislikes have the strongest control over what we eat. We eat what we like based on experience and, unfortunately, most people have little experience with foods that are not part of their typical diet. This makes dieting difficult since preferences for foods are established primarily through learning and experience. In fact, the only genetically based factors in food preferences are people's likes for salty and sweet tastes and dislikes for those that are sour and bitter. Even these unlearned factors can be modified by experience—in fact, *all* preferences (likes) and aversions (dislikes) for foods can be modified.

Yet, to begin to understand why we eat what we eat, it is important first to get an idea of why we diet. After all, dieting typically involves eating foods and flavors different from those we have learned to like. In other words, dieting is in many ways counterintuitive. It often requires us to eat what we do not like, which all but guarantees long-term failure. While there are many reasons for dieting, let's look at just a few.

We diet to appease societal expectations of body image. Billboards display beautiful women who are far thinner than the average healthy American. This kind of image comes before adults, but also before children—who often are brought into the mindset of dieting, and who view an estimated 40,000 advertisements per year on television alone. These include commercials for sugared breakfast cereals, pitches for high-calorie snacks, and alcoholic beverage ads that feature animated characters. Children are also confronted with the contradiction of seeing fast-food ads on educational television in schools, and magazine ads with stick-thin models.[2] We have created a culture that scolds its people for being fat, and then promotes the consumption of the very foods (and drugs) that are making them fat.

More recently, controversy has brewed over a report that at least 59 of the nation's 250 children's hospitals have fast-food restaurants on the premises.[3] What kind of message does that send to kids: "Obesity kills—oh, by the way, if you're hungry there's a McDonald's just down the hall." Conflicting messages make it difficult to address the problem. Businesses such as Hooters and Heart Attack Grill employ beautiful waitresses and have them serve in sexy outfits or in sleek nurse-type uniforms. While not likely the intention of these eateries, this has the effect of lowering self-image among many women and raising expectations of body image to unrealistic proportions. And it doesn't stop there. Image seems to drive most dieters today. People diet because it is the fad or "in" diet, or to attract partners, or to facilitate intimacy and social inclusion, or for all of these reasons. Dieters (especially younger people) aim to lose weight as much to improve how they appear to others as to themselves. Although clear evidence shows that image is not the only reason people diet,[4] we are still largely failing as a society to promote health while succeeding in the promotion of body image.

We diet on impulse. Enter Oprah Winfrey, one of the most accomplished and influential women in world history, and this is no overstatement. When Oprah likes something—anything—so do her adoring fans. Her book club all but guarantees hundreds of thousands of sales of the books she endorses. When she endorses people, they become famous too. Just ask another daytime television personality, Dr. Phil McGraw, who owes much of his success to appearances he made on her show. Her viewers will even subscribe to dieting if she gives the OK. Following a 2006 appearance by authors Mehmet Oz and Michael Roizen on Oprah's television talk show, their dieting books occupied the top three spots on the best-seller list of Amazon.com. Customers were buying the book she endorsed, as well as the DVD version and hardcover editions of the authors' previous work—with total sales exceeding one million dollars, thanks in large part to Oprah.[5] And there you have it—the *dieters' impulse*. Within a week of Oz and Roizen appearing on her show, their books became the standard for dieting, with hundreds of thousands of Oprah Winfrey fans subscribing to a regimen they had likely never heard of before.

This is not the only example, of course. Dieters notoriously go for quick fixes, e.g., to slim down for a prom or wedding, to impress an ex-lover, to fit into a smaller swimsuit before going to the beach, or to keep a significant other satisfied. The point is that the initial goal of a diet is typically short-term. There are immediate reasons (both sacred and secular) for dieting. Rarely does much thought go into choosing a diet; it is simply a decision to lose weight with no apparent concern for what happens after we have reached a goal. One can begin to understand why most diets fail eventually: few dieters set long-term goals.

We do not diet for health. While these reasons do not fully encompass why people diet, one thing is certain: people generally begin dieting for health-related reasons only when health becomes an issue, e.g., when they are older or have experienced a trauma or illness. Sadly, while most diets will drop the pounds, many of them do so at the expense of health. Researchers simply do not know the long-term health consequences of popular diets such as Adkins or South Beach, because these diets have not been around long. Yet that doesn't seem to matter to most people. Dieting is such a social phenomenon that the best reason for being on a diet is lost: to live a longer, healthier life. Unfortunately, health has become a secondary concern for many dieters. With ever-increasing human life expectancies and improvements in health care, drug synthesis, and plastic surgery, this is no wonder. After all, while obesity and eating disorder prevalence has soared in America, so also has the human life expectancy—it has more than doubled in the past century. Therefore, we must return to the beginning to understand why health is so important both in terms of the individual and in terms of the costs associated with unhealthy eating.

A Brief History of Diet

It terms of man's evolution, much of our success can be attributed to our ability to obtain, develop, store, and consume a wide range of foods. Yet, how has this affected our health? Changes in our diet over the past few hundred years include increased intake of saturated fats, refined carbohydrates (CHO), and sodium, and decreased intake of nonnutrient fibers. These changes have likely contributed to the problems overwhelming our healthcare systems. While the utilization of a wide variety of foods has been key to man's survival, recent fad diets have emphasized single food items or nutrients. These diets, even though successful in taking off pounds, are associated with health complications. Restriction to only a few staple foods is a poor-quality diet and generally leads to a decline in health. For example, many researchers believe that high-protein diets will lead to kidney failure.[6,7] Vegetarian diets, such as those that emphasize high soy intake, have been associated with enlargement of the pancreas[8] and iron deficiencies.[9]

Still, variety is not always a good thing. When people are allowed to choose from a variety of foods, they tend to consume more of those foods they like, which tend to be high in sodium, saturated fat, refined CHO, and sugars; i.e., they tend to be unhealthy food options. This was true as much for our ancestors as it is for humans today. An estimated 95% of the dietary intake of our earliest ancestors was in the form of plant foods such as fruits, leaves, gums, and stalks.[10] This means that protein (mostly from vegetable sources) composed the greatest proportion of their diet. Simple CHO intake would be less than today and come mainly from fruits. Dietary fiber intake would be much greater than today and would have contributed to significantly greater daily energy intake. In fact, fiber consumption today is lower than at any other point in our evolution. In general, daily intake of vitamins would have been significantly greater than today. Depending on geographic location, sodium would have been scarce, and likely contributed only a fraction of early ancestral diets. Total fat intake, particularly saturated fats (the "bad" fats), and cholesterol intake would have been significantly below current levels of consumption.[11]

There is consistent evidence that as the human diet continued to shift, there was a gradual decline in the nutritional value of foods consumed. Today, humans are the only free-living mammalian species that ordinarily consumes more sodium than potassium, with about 90% of current sodium intake coming from food processing, preparation, and flavoring. Our early ancestors did not have such unprecedented access to sodium, and also did not experience rising average blood pressure with increasing age, nor did they commonly develop hypertension, as is uniquely characteristic of today's human population.

Cereal grains, especially corn, have replaced fruits and vegetables as our primary source of calories and contribute up to 90% of our daily caloric requirements. Unfortunately, while fruits and vegetables have preventive effects for a variety of cancers, cereal grains have none; if anything, cereal grains have been shown to increase risks for some forms of cancer.[12] Also, cholesterol-raising saturated fats constitute 15% of dietary energy today, compared with 5% for ancestral humans.[13] Moreover, serum cholesterol levels have nearly doubled compared with our hunter-gatherer ancestors and they are highest today in affluent Western societies where coronary heart disease (CHD) is the leading cause of mortality.

So what does all of this mean? It means we have an eating dilemma. The nutritional values of our diets have changed, and not for the better. We do not eat the same foods, or the same quality of foods, as our ancestors did. And while our life expectancies have soared in the past century, so has the prevalence of deadly conditions such as heart disease, stroke, cancer, anorexia, bulimia, depression, and diabetes—all of which are linked to what we eat. Medicines may be keeping us alive longer, but that does not mean we are necessarily healthier— this has been largely evident even over only the past 30 years.

Health in America Today

So what are the health issues facing America today? Well, let's begin with obesity. Obesity is a multifactor disease; it is long-term, and requires long-term treatments. Today, the Body Mass Index (BMI) is used to classify overweight (BMI 25.0-29.9) and obesity (BMI at least 30.0) among adults (age 20 years and over), by calculating height, weight, and gender; notably, this measure does not consider body fat percentage, which is a factor also related to many of the health issues associated with obesity. Obesity is a widespread problem around the globe, termed *Globesity* in a 2006 article describing the rising rates of diabetes, high blood pressure, and obesity in China.[14] The French, known for their low rate of obesity compared with people of other industrialized countries, are also getting fatter.[15] Even in Africa, a region known for malnutrition, obesity is a growing concern, with more than one-third of black women and one-quarter of black men estimated to be overweight.[16] The World Health Organization predicts these statistics will rise substantially in the next 10 years. As of 2005, about 59% of Americans were classified as overweight or obese, with almost a quarter of the American population classified as obese.

The economic costs of obesity are estimated at over 39 billion dollars a year. This includes the costs associated with dieting, prevention, advertising, and unemployment related to obesity, as well as obesity-related medical care and other factors. Although genetic or acquired differences in metabolism play a significant role in obesity, this disease has much to do with learning. Children are told to "clean up your plate" and are praised for doing so, punished when they don't. They are rewarded for eating a healthy meal by being given a high-fat dessert, and (as will be discussed in later chapters) this reinforcement only increases a child's liking for the dessert, not for the healthy meal. Inexpensive, good-tasting, high-fat foods are readily available, whereas healthier foods cost more and are not as widely sold at the drive-through or the snack machine.

The prevalence of malnourished and underweight persons in this country is also staggering.[17] Anorexia nervosa, characterized by severe under eating, even to the point of starvation, can include episodes of bulimia and sometimes leads to suicide. Bulimia nervosa is characterized by loss of control of food intake, and involves periodic eating binges (especially with snacks and desserts), followed by self-induced vomiting or use of laxatives. Because of binging and purging, net nutrient intake can vary widely. Only 19% of bulimics are estimated to actually under eat. Both anorexia and bulimia are most prominent in adolescent women, with bulimia nervosa being more common.

Treatments for these diseases have brought little in the way of positive results. Social and societal factors undoubtedly play large roles, and these most likely interfere with the effectiveness of social therapies. After 20 years of interventions, only 29% of patients have shown good recovery, while almost 15% have committed suicide or died from complications of the disease. Drug therapies have been just as ineffective. Most drugs used to treat these diseases have been targeted at stimulating appetite, and are likely ineffective because anorexics *are* physiologically responsive to food. They don't lack appetite per se; they simply don't act on it.

What of other diseases that arise from unhealthy eating?[18] More than 460 persons per 100,000 were suffering with cancer as of 2002, with males showing higher fatality rates than females. A significant incidence of cancer is undoubtedly linked to diet. The prevalence of diabetes in the United States has nearly tripled in the last 25 years, with at least 25 out of every 100,000 diabetics dying from the disease each year, as of 2005. Still, these figures are dwarfed by the 53 out of every 100,000 persons expected to die of strokes each year and the 232 out of every 100,000 persons expected to die of heart disease each year. The fact is that eating is more than a matter of health; it is a matter of life. Disorders and diseases almost non-existent in previous generations are now among the leading causes of human death!

The Dieting Dilemma

The human diet has expanded. Survival is no longer a matter of eating enough; it is a matter of eating right. It is not the volume of food consumed that makes us fatter, as much as it is the healthfulness of those foods. In other words, healthy eating is more than counting calories; it is counting where those calories come from. Yet for many people, the "healthy calories" come from foods that don't taste very good, such as the bitter tasting vegetables or sour tasting fruits. In order to begin eating healthy we must do more than just start eating healthier foods; we must learn to like them as well. The problem is that changing our diets is genuinely easier said than done. Just ask the majority of dieters who are unable to remain on healthier diets—anyone can change their diet, but few can truly make these changes long-term.

What this means is that we find ourselves in a dieting dilemma. The weight loss equation seems simple enough: if *calories in* are less than *calories out,* then body fat will decrease. Of course, dieting is much more complex than this. It is unfortunate that the term "diet" has come to mean connotatively something negative. A dieter is looked upon as someone who already has a weight or eating problem—why else would the person be dieting? But dieting should be more than that. All people (healthy or not) diet—after all, a diet is basically characterized by the foods one consumes to survive, regardless of how those foods affect health or figure. It is also apparent that many dieters could use a change in their diets—just read through the statistics again if you are not convinced. Yet while all dieters should consume healthier foods every day as part of a regular diet, many don't. What this book teaches is the psychology of why we eat the foods we eat—even if they kill us. In all, this book reviews a vast literature from many areas of psychology to explain how we learn about the foods we eat and how we can apply this learning to improve the health of our diets long-term.

It is also important to note that many books, nutritionists, and resources are available on healthy eating. What is healthy for one person may not be healthy for another. A person with diabetes will require a different diet from a person suffering from thyroid deficiency, and a person who just suffered a heart attack will need a different diet from a healthy individual. Age, health status, weight, gender, ethnicity, socioeconomic status, and many other factors play roles in determining what foods are apart of your diet and what makes that diet nutritious. One diet does not fit all, and those who claim otherwise are trying to sell you something. This book does not tell you what diet you should go on, because no one diet will work for everyone. Instead, this book teaches about the psychology behind why we eat, why we like what we eat, and how to enjoy consuming a healthier diet long-term. This is your health, your lifestyle, and your quality of life. Find a healthier diet that works for you, and this book will provide you with the psychological know-how to make it a success.

Gregory J. Privitera, Ph.D.
Glendale, Arizona
September, 2007

Notes

1. Jeffery, R. W., Epstein, L. H., Wilson, G. T., Drewnowski, A., Stunkard, A. J., & Wing, R. R. (2000). Long-term maintenance of weight loss: Current status. *Health Psychology*, 19 (1S), 5-16.
2. Reported online by the Associated Press: "Study: Fast food in kids' hospitals sends mixed message," 12 Dec 2006.
3. Reported online by the Associated Press: "Ads spur eating disorders, premature drinking, docs say," 4 Dec 2006.
4. Ziegler, P. J., Khoo, C. S., Sherr, B., Nelson, J. A., Larson, W. M., & Drewnowski, A. (1998). Body image and dieting behaviors among elite figure skaters. *International Journal of Eating Disorders*, 24 (4), 421-427.
5. Reported online by the Associated Press: "Oprah's nod makes diet books a hit," 6 Nov 2006.
6. Hammond, K.A., & Janes, D.N. (1998). The effects of increased protein intake on kidney size and function. *J. Exp. Biol.*, 201, 2081-2090.
7. Klahr, S. (1989). Effects of protein intake on the progression of renal disease. *Ann. Rev. Nutr.*, 9, 87-108.
8. Liener, I.E. (1994). Implications of antinutritional components of soybean foods. *Crit. Rev. Food Sci. Nutr.*, 34, 31-67.
9. Shaw, N.S., Chin, C.J., & Pan, W.H. (1995). A vegetarian diet rich in soy bean products compromises iron status in young students. *J. Nutr.*, 125, 212-219.

10. Milton, K. (1993). Diet and primate evolution. *Sci. Am., 269*, 86-93.
11. For review see Ungar, P.S. & Teaford, M. F. (2002). *Human diet: Its origin and evolution.* Westport, CT: Greenwood Publishing, Inc.
12. World Cancer Research Fund and American Institute for Cancer Research (1997). *Food, nutrition, and the prevention of cancer: A global perspective* (pp. 506-507). Washington, D.C.: American Institute for Cancer Research.
13. Eaton, S.B.; Eaton, S.B. III, & Konner, M.J. (1997). Paleolithic nutrition revisited: A twelve-year retrospective on its nature and implications. *Eur. J. Clin. Nutr., 51*, 207-216.
14. Reported online by the Associated Press: "Globesity: 60 million Chinese are obese," 6 Nov 2006.
15. Reported online by the Associated Press: "The French are getting fatter and taller, study says," 2 Feb 2007.
16. Reported online by the Associated Press: "Africa faces growing obesity problem," 29 Nov 2006.
17. For review, see Carlson, N.R. (2001). *Physiology and Behavior*, 8th Ed. (pp. 392-422). Boston, MA: Allyn & Bacon Publishing.
18. Statistics reported in this paragraph were taken from the Henry J. Kaiser Family Foundation website: http://statehealthfacts.org.

SECTION I: Why We Feel Hungry and Full

Chapter 1: Monitoring Calories

On a dreary, rainy morning in our nation's capital, my dad and I began our trek in the 26.2-mile, 22nd annual Marine Corps Marathon. More than 19,000 athletes from around the globe *paid a fee* to run, walk, bike, jog, Rollerblade, and even march in formation along the picturesque streets of Washington, D.C. The participants were all smiles as we crossed the starting line. You could hear people asking in sarcastic tones the age-old questions such as, "Water stops— who needs those?" and, "How far is this race again?" It didn't take a psychologist to observe the sarcasm fading quickly into concerns such as, "How much farther till the next water stop?" and, "How is it that I've run 15 miles and still have over 10 to go?" It is interesting that as the race goes on, people's concerns become more rudimentary. Participants count the miles down as if they have come too far to quit. Food and water become the topics of the day as some people talk about their favorite foods while others, too tired to talk, just listen and drool. Many runners were looking for food stops as the race was taking its toll. My dad and I didn't need food stops (or so we thought), because we strategically placed jellybeans (for sugar energy) into convenient little pockets in our running shorts. We bragged to each other that we had outsmarted them all! Of course what we didn't count on was running out of jellybeans: as we crossed the 22nd mile marker that is exactly what happened.

We passed a group of friendly spectators handing out PowerBars—I hated PowerBars! The bitter taste and bland flavor didn't sit well with my taste buds, but what choice did I have? I was running out of energy, and my dad was urging me to take some. I needed something to get me through the last leg of this race, and I really had no fight left in me to disagree. So, taking my dad's advice, and with some reluctance, I took a piece of the PowerBar and ate it. To my utter surprise, it tasted delicious! The taste rivaled my preference for any Italian dish I can think of (and I love Italian). The bar couldn't have tasted better. I took more, and soon found myself in an energy-packed paradise. I had finally discovered the great taste of a dietary nutrition bar. With each bite, I found myself wanting more, finally appreciating the culinary contribution of this nutritious energy bar. Right there, at the 22nd mile of the 22nd annual Marine Corps Marathon, I loved it! It was better than a slice of homemade apple pie; more satisfying than a tall glass of lemonade on a hot summer day; it tasted like heaven! Although far from satiated, my father and I felt as if we had enough energy to take on the world as we crossed that elusive finish line—in under four hours.

A week later, I was looking for a quick fix for lunch and came across a small shop. There on the shelves behind the cashier was my newfound love—PowerBars in all sorts of great flavors including chocolate. I immediately bought one; being as though I was still sore from my marathon, it made sense that I should fill up with nutrition. I opened it and took a much-anticipated bite, and something strange happened. To my dismay, my newfound liking had disappeared. I spit out the bar as fast as it had entered my mouth! The taste was horrible—but how could this be? I loved the taste of it only a week earlier. Then, I couldn't get enough of the nutrition bar. I would have bought an entire store's supply of the stuff at the 22nd mile of that marathon, but now I couldn't bear even to look at it. How did my preference shift from liking to disliking in just a week? It was an answer that would take me years to learn and one that emphasizes a main theme of this book: *what we like and choose to eat is largely the result of learning, and what is learned can be modified.*

As it turns out, the answer is that a person's liking for the flavors they consume is more pronounced when his or her body is deprived of food or water.[1,2] It is likely that if I had tasted that same bar at the second mile of the marathon, I would have readily rejected it. Instead, I consumed the bar toward the end of the race, a point at which my deprivation of food and water was great, and so I liked it—if only for a moment. This is a wonderful mechanism for liking. We eat what we like; therefore, it would be advantageous to like foods (even the foods we dislike) when we are in great need of the energy they provide.

Naturally, I hope this account doesn't motivate parents to deprive their kids of food or force them to run marathons in order to get them to eat their vegetables; there are other, more practical ways to do that, which I will mention in this book. What I hope the reader can understand from this introduction is that *why we eat* and *why we like* are connected, but distinct. For example, I ate the energy bar because I was deprived of calories; i.e., I was deprived of energy. But I also liked the taste because I was deprived—a taste that I would otherwise not prefer (and still do not like). What is perplexing is that my liking for this bar ceased as soon as my deprivation ceased. Liking for food that we do not like seems to be short-term, but that is because we fail to understand what causes liking. For example, as an infantryman in the U.S. Marines, I would consume Meals-Ready-To-Eat (MREs) during training exercises. These are prepackaged foods, sealed in airtight packaging and stored for years until they are consumed. While these meals are packed with nutrition, they aren't readily available on your grocers' shelves for good reasons: they are expensive, and they aren't very appetizing. But don't tell that to a U.S. Marine, including me—as the saying goes: once a Marine, always a Marine. In the field, Marines are regularly deprived of basic necessities, so when these needs are met, they are appreciated. I consumed these nutrient-packed meals two or three times a day under high deprivation, usually following long and tedious exercises. While I initially disliked them, over time that began to change—I began to enjoy them. I would even eat them back in the comforts of my own barracks, where I had alternative choices for a meal and was not necessarily deprived when I consumed them. In other words, I was no longer dependent on deprivation to enjoy a food I would otherwise have rejected.

Consider also just some of the psychology in the culinary choices we make—why do we eat when we are *not* hungry? Why do we prefer some foods to others? Why do we avoid foods that are new to us? If we have only one bad experience with a food, why do we go out of our way to avoid eating that food again? Why do many people prefer unhealthy foods? Why is there "room" for dessert, even when we feel full? There is no question that physiological factors play an essential role in our choices and attitudes in regard to foods. Still, in order to understand *why we eat* and *why we like*, it is important to look first at the physiological factors involved in the appetizing decisions we make. After all, one thing is certain: we must eat to live.

Homeostasis

Early psychological research on eating behaviors focused primarily on the physiological mechanisms involved. In the late nineteenth century, the distinguished researcher Claude Bernard found that the body actively maintains the constancy of its internal environment.[3] Early physiological psychologists were interested in finding the internal cue that initiated eating (hunger cue) and the internal cue that ceased eating (satiety cue). Researchers initially hypothesized a *wisdom of the body* whereby these internal cues signal some physiological need (such as a need for sugar), thus producing a desire to fulfill that need (such as craving a candy bar). This view was the primary focus from the 1930s to the 1950s for researchers seeking knowledge about what is now referred to as a homeostatic system.

Walter Cannon, who was among the first to use the term "homeostasis" in his 1932 book, appropriately titled *The Wisdom of the Body*, defined it as a tendency to uniformity or stability in the normal body states of an organism with compensatory mechanisms to preserve constancy.[4] Stated more simply, homeostasis is a change in the face of change so as to remain unchanged. Many functions in our body are regulated by a homeostatic system. For example, we appear to maintain a constant body weight over time. The body regulates this ultimately by increasing how much we eat when our body weight is too low and decreasing our intake when it is too high. Temperature is also regulated by a homeostatic system. Average body temperature is 98.6° Fahrenheit, but a person's body isn't always at this temperature. Instead, the body allows its temperature to fluctuate within a range that keeps the person healthy. Thus when temperature changes, so does this system, in order to keep the body temperature as unchanged as possible.

The introduction of the idea of homeostasis sparked wide interest across many disciplines of psychology. Its popularity grew such that researchers were using this newly defined phenomenon to describe and explain principles such as perception, reasoning, rationalization, and personality. At the time that the idea became widespread, the drive to maintain an internal balance was considered one of the most powerful of biological urges. One of the most recognized advocates of the power of biological drives was Clark Hull, whose drive-reduction theory[5] has lost favor as a satisfactory explanation for eating behaviors within recent decades. He believed that we eat to reduce a drive (e.g., hunger). He defined all behavior essentially as being driven, such that all behavior acts to reduce drives. This theory, though, has many shortcomings, including the fact that drives—the basis for his theory—are merely *hypothetical constructs*. Unless we define "drives," they don't really exist, since they can't be directly observed. Also, not all behaviors reduce a physiological need or drive: we are motivated to eat even when we are not hungry, and we eat even when we feel full.

Around the time of Hull's work, an equally interesting explanation for food selection was surfacing; one that emphasized that food selection was dependent on gene-determined individual differences.[6] This explanation, introduced by researcher W. F. Dove, paralleled an evolutionary ideology in the sense that according to this logic, genetically superior animals in a group would choose more nutritionally beneficial diets. He referred to these animals as *aggridant types*. These were characterized by superior size, physical form, rate of reproduction, and longevity of life. All of these paralleled Darwinian characterizations of dominant members within species. Charles Darwin himself—as author of the theory of evolution[7]—might have described such characteristics in terms of fitness. Yet, although genetics have a large impact on the foods we choose to consume, you will see that the influence of genetics pertains primarily to the foods and flavors we eventually prefer, and our predisposed tendencies to prefer these flavorful foods are not entirely dependent on their nutritional content.

Nutritionists in the 1940s generally agreed that the intake of adequate nutrition was important for health, and that the purpose of meeting nutritional requirements was to prevent the appearance of negative symptoms associated with unhealthy eating, such as weight gain. In a review article in 1948, researcher P. T. Young wrote that the psychology of such a perspective must link nutritional requirements to behavior. He noticed that learning, experience, and the palatability (or pleasantness) of foods were all variables that affected the food-seeking behaviors he observed in his laboratories. In other words, factors not directly related to the number of calories we consume could affect what and how much we eat. Therefore, for homeostasis to be a primary factor it was important to link a change in homeostatic balance (such as a deprivation in some nutritional need) with the behaviors associated with "correcting" the homeostatic unbalance (such as seeking water, shade, rest, or food).[8] He insisted that while dietary need is a nutritional concept, we do not eat only because we need nutrition. Instead, he viewed drives as more of a measuring tool than an overt behavior. This was a rather unconventional perspective in the 1940s; theorists at the time were more focused on the physiological components of eating and considered drives to be "preprogrammed" behavioral responses to physiological needs such as hunger. This critical review put forward the possibility that we do not eat simply to satisfy a homoeostatic need. It also reflected the changing focus that researchers would take many decades later.

As we crossed into the second half of the twentieth century, two influential theories arose as an attempt to clarify the functional role of a homeostatic system for eating behaviors. These theories, known as the glucostatic[9] and the lipostatic[10] theories of feeding regulation, explained the internal signals and cues that were involved in maintaining a homeostatic balance. Yet, although these theories explained the model well, the model itself was rather limiting in its application to all eating behaviors. In the late 1950s and into the 1960s, researchers discovered many fundamental flaws with the homeostatic model.

The Secondary Role of Learning

Learning plays a secondary role in the homeostatic model. The model assumes essentially that we learn where food is, but we won't go there and eat it until we are hungry. The diminished role that learning plays in this model limits its application to eating behavior. Consider the reality of a body that can seek food only when it is deprived or hungry. What if no food was available? How would you be able to replenish your glucose, amino acids, lipids, and other nutritional requirements that are obviously depleted? It would indubitably be advantageous to eat in anticipation of being hungry or thirsty, (say) by eating a small snack to hold you over until dinner, even if you are not that hungry, or by drinking a liter of water before a long run, even when you are not thirsty. Researchers recognized a simple fact: humans eat and drink not only in *response* to hunger and thirst, but also in *anticipation* of them. The homeostatic model gave credence to the idea that humans learn where food is (such as in a refrigerator), but do not act on that knowledge until they are hungry. I'm sure you don't need to think too hard to remember a time that you ate when you were not hungry. Many desserts have found their way into my belly well after I was satiated and well before I was hungry. Instead, learning actually plays a primary role in determining what we eat, when we eat it, and whether we like what we eat.

Have you ever packed a lunch before heading to work in the morning? Do you prepare the Thanksgiving turkey hours prior to dinner? Do you shop for several days' worth of groceries at a time, or just for the next meal? These are simple and practical examples of how we learn about food. We are seldom surprised by the expectation that we will eat a meal, or by its timing. We fully expect to eat, and we prepare food in the oven or microwave or on the stove in anticipation of eating later. We aren't necessarily hungry at the time we are cooking. We are fully aware that not eating for a while makes us feel like eating, so why wait until that uncomfortable moment to begin preparation when we can anticipate it?

The night prior to running the marathon, my dad and I drank over six liters of water and consumed a large portion of a carbohydrate-dense meal of spaghetti. Why? Well, we were about to run a 26.2-mile marathon. Anticipating that we would need the energy was common sense to us, as I hope it was to the rest of the runners. That is the point: if we can anticipate the need to feed, then learning must play a primary role in the formulation of our diets. While an unconditioned event, such as a homeostatic signal to consume food, does not need to be learned, the anticipation of such events *does* require learning. The message, as unconventional as it may seem, is to *stop counting the calories and start counting where the calories are coming from*. While we do not need to learn to consume calories (this is the energy a homeostatic system monitors), we do need to learn where to get those calories and which foods to get them from. Thus, the major components of our diets are learned. This is good news, since what is learned can be modified through experience.

The Primary Role of Hunger and Satiety

The development of eating patterns, likes, dislikes, and digestive responses is subject to learning. Eating patterns pertain to the number of meals you eat each day, what types of foods are characteristically part of your diet, the size of your meals, and so on. Yet, if hunger and satiety were the main factors that cause eating, how would we learn to like some foods and not others? How would we select among different diets? For example, in the 1960s, researcher Paul Rozin showed that thiamine-deficient rats will choose a thiamine-rich diet when allowed to choose freely among four different meals, only one of which contained thiamine.[11] The thiamine-deficient rats in Paul Rozin's experiment *learned* that the three thiamine-depleted diets left them feeling ill, while the thiamine-rich diet did not. Thus, the rats *learned* which diet to consume based on the *consequences* of their eating behavior. Learning played a primary role in diet selection.

You may be wondering why we should care about the diet selection of rats. Well, healthy rats characteristically follow random feeding patterns that consist of sampling small amounts of different novel (or "new") foods at first. This is similar to a child's feeding pattern—most parents understand that getting children to eat new foods is no simple task. After tasting a new food, rats usually will continue to eat that food, so long as they don't become sick—presumably because they now consider it safe to eat. What makes rats a unique subject for testing is that they have essentially co-evolved with humans. Rats have eaten of human scraps for presumably as long as humans have existed. This makes them ideal subjects in laboratory experiments, since they will eat foods similar to those that we enjoy. In fact, much of what we know about human feeding today, we first learned in rats.

Studies conducted by Ivan Pavlov as far back as the 1920s presented evidence that digestive processes could be altered through experience.[12] Unfortunately, this evidence was not empirically recognized for decades. Pavlov, who is probably better known for his research on classical conditioning than for his Nobel Prize-winning research on digestion, found that dogs salivate more or less according to the kind of food used in the experiment. As dogs learned which foods were harder to swallow than others, they also learned to salivate more in anticipation of having to digest the more difficult foods. This realization, that *involuntary* physiological responses such as salivation could be altered through experience, challenged how encompassing a homeostatic model could be in explaining all aspects of eating behaviors. After all, if involuntary reflexes can be subject to learning, then homeostatic regulation should be subject to learning.

As it turns out, homeostatic systems *are* subject to learning. For instance, when we eat, the level of glucose (a usable form of caloric energy) rises in the bloodstream. When this rise is detected, the pancreas produces insulin, which enters the bloodstream and starts essentially to store the glucose we consume. If insulin levels rise before glucose gets in the bloodstream, then we won't have enough glucose for energy (referred to as hypoglycemic). If insulin levels drop too low, then we will have too much glucose in the bloodstream (referred to as hyperglycemic). Contrary to the predictions of a homeostatic model, this metabolic process (which regulates the glucose available in the bloodstream) is subject to learning: insulin not only responds to the energy we consume, but also to stimuli that predict the energy.

In one study, Woods and colleagues found that through learning, cues associated with foods that increase blood glucose could come to elicit insulin secretion prematurely (referred to as *cephalic insulin*). These researchers conditioned rats to be hypoglycemic—to have low blood glucose levels.[13] Rodents were presented with a tone (the conditioned cue) prior to a dessert food (an unconditioned cue, which increases blood glucose levels, thereby increasing the amount of insulin in the blood). After several pairings, the tone elicited an increase in insulin even when the food was not presented. This insulin release in the absence of the food (i.e., in the absence of glucose) caused low blood glucose levels or hypoglycemia. These researchers were also able to cause conditioned hyperglycemia—high blood glucose levels.[14] Rodents were given the same tone-food pairings that were used in their previous work, but in this case the researchers removed the tone after training; i.e., they presented the food alone without the tone preceding it. The result was a delay in the secretion of insulin formerly predicted by the tone, temporarily causing high blood glucose levels or hyperglycemia.

If insulin secretion into the bloodstream were strictly homeostatic, then insulin should only be released in *response* to energy intake, and yet it also *anticipates* energy intake (i.e., insulin secretion can be modified by learning). Because of the complexities of human feeding and the readily available groceries in supermarkets worldwide, the homeostatic system, which itself is subject to learning, likely plays only a minor role in the control of feeding in today's food-rich society. There are simply too many cues associated with feeding for physiological disturbances to play a primary role in the formulation of human diet.

We Do Not Eat Only Because We Are Hungry

Learning doesn't depend on hunger or on some state of deficiency, as implied by the homeostatic model. Researchers, for example, have repeatedly shown that animals learn to respond to nutritionally useless foods, such as saccharin—which tastes sweet but has no appreciable nutritional value. In a homeostatic model, the deprivations initiating hunger are always physiological. Therefore, if only physiological deprivations initiate hunger, saccharin should never be reinforcing, since it does not contain the nutrients necessary to meet these physiological needs. Contrary to the model, saccharin-sweetened water has been shown to be preferred by rats over plain water,[15] and more current research has successfully used saccharin as a reinforcer to reverse *innate* (or unlearned) preferences, resulting in a preference for a sour taste (i.e., citric acid) over a salty taste.[16] So rats are motivated to consume a nutrient-depleted solution, but are humans?

Yes, products such as Equal sweetener are used to enhance the taste and liking for foods, but contain no appreciable calories. What is more is that humans do not entirely judge fullness and hunger on calories consumed either. How much we eat and when we eat are controlled in large part by other learned factors including the time of day, how good the food tastes or smells, a clock ("It's time to eat"), the sight of food, or whether other persons are eating. Generally, how much other people eat is an implicit social norm—"I can have seconds since everyone else is." Researcher Barbara Rolls recently demonstrated that a liquid food can be depleted of half its calories and we are none the wiser.[17] Subjects judged fullness on how much they ate of a food, even if that food contained half the calories. The likelihood is that if I took up to half the calories out of your diet but allowed you to consume the same amount of food, you might not notice the difference.

So, do we eat because we are hungry? Yes, but even hunger is susceptible to learning. Indeed, it may be just as common for people to eat when they are *not* hungry. The take away message is that hunger and fullness are influenced by more than just the calories we consume. In many ways, our psychology has stronger control over what foods we eat (and how much we eat) than our physiology. Interestingly, one of the strongest predictors of what foods we like is the experience that comes with age.[18] Thus, what foods we like and select to eat depend in large part on our experiences with (or learning about) different foods, and not entirely on an innate biological process. If we preferred healthier food options, we would make them available for consumption; but, unfortunately, many people don't. This means that simply counting calories is not a solution for improving the health of our diets. This will be emphasized throughout the book.

Notes

1. Capaldi, E. D. (1982). Taste preferences as a function of food deprivation during original taste exposure. *Animal Learning & Behavior*, 10 (2), 211-219.
2. Revusky, S.H. (1967). Hunger level during food consumption: Effects on subsequent preference. *Psychonomic Science, 7*, 109-110.
3. Bernard, C. (1878). *Lecons sur les phénomènes de la vie communs aux animaux et aux végétaux* [Lessons on the phenomena of the life common to the animals and to plants]. Paris: J. B. Bailliere.
4. Cannon, W. B. (1932). *The Wisdom of the Body*. New York: Norton.
5. Hull, C.L. (1943). *Principles of behavior*. New York: Appleton.
6. Dove, W. F. (1939). The needs of superior individuals as guides to group ascendance. *Journal of Heredity, 30*, 157-163.
7. Darwin, C. (1979). *The Origin of Species* (reprint). New York: Gramercy Books.
8. Young, P. T. (1948). Appetite, palatability and feeding habit: a critical review. *Psychological Bulletin, 45*, 289-320.
9. Mayer, J. (1953). Glucostatic mechanisms of regulation of food intake. *New England Journal of Medicine, 249*, 13-16.
10. Kennedy, G. C. (1950). The hypothalamic control of food intake in rats. *Proceedings of the Royal Society of London, 137B*, 535-548.
11. Rozin, P. (1969). Adaptive food sampling patterns in vitamin deficient rats. *Journal of Comparative and Physiological Psychology, 76* (3), 126-132.
12. Pavlov, I. P. (1927). *Conditioned Reflexes*. Oxford, England: Oxford University Press.
13. Woods, S. C. (1976). Conditioned hypoglycemia. *Journal of Comparative and Physiological Psychology, 90*, 1164-1168.
14. Woods, S. C. (1977). Conditioned insulin secretion. In Y. Katsuk, M. Sato, S. I. Takagi, & Y. Oomura (Eds.), *Food Intake and the Chemical Senses* (pp. 331-342). Tokyo: University of Tokyo Press.
15. Mook, D. G. (1974). Saccharin preference in the rat: Some unpalatable findings. *Psychological Review, 81* (6), 475-490.
16. Capaldi, E. D., Hunter, M. J., & Lyn, S. A. (1997). Conditioning with taste as the CS in conditioned flavor preference learning. *Animal Learning & Behavior*, 25 (4), 427-436.
17. Bell, E. A., Roe, L. S., & Rolls, B. J. (2003). Sensory-specific satiety is affected more by volume than by energy content of a liquid food. *Physiology & Behavior*, 78 (4-5), 593-600.
18. Drewnowski, A., Henderson, S. A., Hann, C. S., Barratt-Fornell, A., & Ruffin, M. (1999). Age and food preferences influence dietary intakes of breast care patients. *Health Psychology*, 18 (6), 570-578.

Chapter 2: Storing and Using Calories

Metabolism is the process by which the body uses and stores the energy we consume (measured in calories). The energy we consume includes nutrients such as carbohydrates, fats, proteins, and sugars, all of which are used by the cells in our body to stay healthy and function properly. Our metabolism stores and uses energy daily and plays a significant role in maintaining short-term body weight through two alternating phases: absorptive and fasting phases. Metabolizing the foods we eat is essential for survival. We must ingest molecules for a variety of nourishing and necessary functions: to construct and maintain our internal organs, to provide our cells with amino acids (the building blocks for life), to provide energy for muscular movements and normal brain functioning, and even to keep our bodies warm. Even shivering requires energy!

Functionally, eating is our way to obtain the energy that is used and stored by our bodies. The foods we eat contain carbohydrates, fats, proteins, and minerals—all of which our body can break down and use to provide energy for our cells. This process of breaking down nutrients is referred to as *digestion* and can take about an hour. If your body has a tendency to store a lot of the nutrients you consume (instead of using them for energy), then you will likely gain weight. So understanding when and why our bodies store nutrients is important to understanding why we gain weight. In a best-case scenario, dieting should involve losing weight, while also allowing our bodies to have the energy they need to function properly. Understanding how metabolism works will help us to do this.

Storing Energy: Spend What You Have and Save the Rest for Later

Our cells are constantly preparing for a worst-case scenario by storing for future needs whatever energy they don't use. You may think of energy storage as a cell's way of opening up a checking or savings account. Many people cash their paychecks, put some in their wallets, some in their checking accounts, and the rest in their savings accounts. The expectation of many of us is that we will spend first from the money we have with us. When that runs out, we take money available to us from our checking accounts. The goal is to steer clear of our savings and use that money only if we must. This is how we spend money and this is how we save money. If we take the old-school approach (before the advent of the credit card), our bodies' energy stores parallel our tendencies toward saving and spending money.

While people need money to acquire the necessities of life, cells likewise need energy. So they use whatever energy they have with them (i.e., energy available in the bloodstream and surrounding cells). This is essentially the cell's wallet. It is the energy that is most readily accessible—the body's "spendable energy," so to speak. But that energy will run out within hours of eating a meal, and cells are constantly competing for this energy. This is when our cells, at least the ones that still need energy, turn to their short-term (checking account) storage of energy. Short-term energy reserves are located in the liver and the muscles. However, muscles are rather selfish with their energy, so most of the energy available to cells in the rest of the body comes from the liver. To store energy, insulin (a peptide hormone produced by the pancreas) converts glucose (a simple sugar) to glycogen (a complex insoluble carbohydrate). This conversion is parallel to converting cash into electronic funds at a bank. Something useful (such as money) is now nothing more than a statement with an account number. Assuming the credit card is not available yet, the only way to make the deposit useful again is to convert it back to money. In the same way, the energy that is stored cannot be used again until it is converted back into glucose. To do this, glucagon (another peptide hormone produced by the pancreas) converts glycogen back into glucose, which enters the bloodstream and is used by cells.

Thus, when the readily available energy is low, our cells begin making transactions in the liver to release more glucose in the bloodstream. These short-term energy stores are useful because they allow our cells to use energy even if we have not eaten for hours. But if we continue not to eat, sooner or later the short-term stores will be depleted, forcing the cells to use long-term stores located in our adipose tissue (i.e., fatty tissues). The average liver can store approximately 300 calories for short-term energy. On the other hand, fatty tissues can store many times more energy. Our adipose tissue consists of cells capable of absorbing nutrients from blood, converting them to triglycerides, and storing them. This is the cells' savings account, reserved for emergencies and used only when necessary. It is these stores that tend to account for a significant proportion of our long-term weight gains and losses.

Generally speaking our metabolism likes to put away energy in our long-term (savings account) storage, same as we would prefer to save money. This is likely why we often do not feel full until we have overeaten. With each meal, our metabolism tries to save energy, and the only way to do this is to eat more than we need, so the amount we don't use can be stored for later. As you will learn in the section titled "Inefficient Metabolism," our metabolisms are seemingly trying to prepare for a famine that isn't likely to happen in our food-rich

Western culture. This helps to explain why we consume more nutrients than we need.

The Phases of Metabolism: A Process of Storing and Using Energy

Absorptive Phase. The absorptive phase begins when we start to eat. In this phase, the food we eat is absorbed and digested so that nutrients can enter the bloodstream and be made available to the cells. As nutrients are absorbed, blood glucose levels rise. The brain, which then initiates parasympathetic activity—generally involved in the storage of excess nutrients—detects this rise. In response, the pancreas stops secreting glucagon and begins secreting insulin, which is used to store the glucose now arriving in the bloodstream. Whatever glucose the cells don't use is converted to glycogen and stored in the liver (short-term stores). When the short-term stores are full, the excess glucose is converted to triglycerides and stored in adipose tissues (long-term stores).

The use of energy during this phase can vary. For the most part, though, amino acids are used either as the building blocks to construct proteins and peptides, or are converted to triglycerides and stored in adipose tissue. Glucose is used mostly by the brain and muscles, with the excess levels being stored in the liver and/or adipose tissues. Fats are not used during the absorptive phase and are stored directly into adipose tissue. This is why one of the most basic ways to lose weight is simply to *decrease the amount of fat you consume in your diet.* Unfortunately, fat tastes great to most people; and what we like, we eat. Also, fat is the most energy-dense nutrient we consume (nine calories per gram, compared with only four in carbohydrates and proteins).

Fasting Phase. The fasting phase begins when the gut is empty, i.e., when the nutrients we consumed have been digested, absorbed, used, and stored. The falling levels of glucose are ultimately detected by the brain, which is alone in being able to use glucose as energy during this phase. The reason is that glucose is water soluble, not lipid (fat) soluble, and therefore cannot pass easily through cell membrane walls since they are constructed of a lipid bi-layer. Therefore cells must have glucose transporters (protein molecules located on the cell membrane) to aid in getting glucose into the cells. However, for most cells outside the brain, these transporters contain insulin receptors. This means that these protein receptors can bring glucose into the cell only if insulin is available and binds with these receptors. On the other hand, transporters on cells in the brain do not contain insulin receptors, which allow glucose to be readily absorbed into cells even when insulin isn't available. This is important because insulin is not available during the fasting phase of metabolism. The fasting phase—triggered by low blood glucose levels—initiates sympathetic activity to break down and utilize the stored nutrients. One way it accomplishes this is to stop producing insulin. The pancreas stops secreting insulin and begins secreting glucagon, which will convert the short-term stores of glycogen back into glucose. This means that (without the presence of insulin) only cells in the brain can use glucose for energy during this phase.

Long-term stores of triglycerides in the adipose tissues are also converted into useful energy, in the forms of glycerol, glucose, and fatty acids. As in the absorptive phase, the use of energy during this phase can vary. Glucose is reserved for use by brain cells. The liver will also covert glycerol (from the adipose tissues) into glucose for energy if needed. Again, without insulin present, only brain cells can use glucose for energy in this phase. The rest of the body, on the other hand, uses the fatty acids from adipose tissue for energy. Fatty acids are metabolized (i.e., used for energy) by all cells in the body except those in the brain, and only in times of fasting. This is why nutritionists emphasize "burning" fats to lose weight, because your body uses fat sparingly and stores it whenever possible.

Inefficient Metabolism: It's Feast or Famine, or at Least it Used to Be

You may have noticed that it seems our metabolism is designed to keep us fat, similar to putting as much into the savings account as possible. That's kind of a smart idea, don't you think? This is, in fact, essentially what our metabolism was designed to do, to maximize the use and storage of the energy we consume. Foraging today involves little more than driving to the local grocery to select and purchase food. Shopping carts are available so you don't have to carry your food, and rarely are any of your foods alive when you purchase them (with the exception of some seafood). On a busy day you may need to push your way through the crowds to grab the last turkey for the Thanksgiving feast but, all in all, foraging is a relatively harmless event today.

Food is readily available, prepackaged, stored at appropriate temperatures, seasoned, grilled, cut thin or thick, bottled, and sealed. The challenges that faced our foraging ancestors—or even those of a few hundred years ago—simply do not exist today. We have the capability to travel the world, drive from state to continental state in a matter of hours, and even forage for food on laptop computers in the comforts of home. Foragers did not have these luxuries. While the developing technology of agriculture has facilitated our ability to store food longer, this is still a recent development. Our evolution (or our genetic adaptation to the environment) takes hundreds of thousands of years. Modern agriculture has existed only a few hundred years. There were times, of course, when foragers hunted without finding food. That would be like going to the supermarket today and finding that everything was sold out—a scenario that is beyond our comprehension. But that was reality for our ancestors. Acquiring food took greater effort, time, and skill. There was no checkout line and there was no guarantee that foraging would produce food. This was once the standard of consumption: a *feast or famine* lifestyle, with limited ability to predict when the feasts or famines would begin and end. This was the environment in which our metabolism evolved and to which it adapted, and this is likely why we store excess energy both short-term and long-term.

You may conclude that this means heavier persons are evolutionarily superior, and to some extent you would be correct. Our metabolism was designed to use energy efficiently. It was designed to use as little energy as possible to perform cellular functions, so the rest of the energy could be stored for the time when famine would come. Our cells don't waste energy. This is one reason why health professionals commonly suggest *not eating within an hour of sleep.* Our cells don't use as much energy during rest (although many of our cells remain active); therefore, much more of the energy (or calories) you consume just prior to sleep will be stored, not used.

So how does one determine the *efficiency* of metabolism? Think of it as if it were fuel for your car. If Car A gets 30 miles to the gallon and Car B gets 40 miles to the gallon, then which car uses fuel more efficiently? It is Car B, because one gallon of fuel in that car provided more output (40 compared with 30 miles per gallon). The more-efficient car used less fuel per mile and left more in the tank. Our metabolism works in a similar way—the efficient metabolism uses less energy to satisfy the needs of our cells. But instead of just leaving the fuel in the tank, so to speak, our bodies store the rest. For example (all other things being equal), assume Jack and Jill each consume a meal containing 500 calories. If Jack requires 450 calories for his cells to perform their daily functions, then only 50 calories will be stored in his liver—recall that the average liver can store approximately 300 calories. On the other hand, Jill's cells require only 200 calories to perform the same functions. In this case Jill's cells use 200 calories of the meal and will store the 300 leftover calories. That would fill up her short-term stores in the liver. Jill has a very efficient metabolism, requiring much fewer calories to do the same job as Jack's cells. Thus, her metabolism gets more miles to the gallon, so to speak—although I doubt she'll be happy about it.

What this also means is that she can't consume as many calories as Jack if she wants to maintain a similar body weight (again, assuming all other factors to be equal). This is one common explanation for the individual differences in how much people can eat without gaining weight. Who would have thought efficiency could be such a bad thing? Bad, that is, if your goal is to lose weight. While evolution will eventually take its course, for now, an efficient metabolism is nothing more than an outdated solution to a new, industrialized, food-rich, *feast and feast some more* existence.

I Can't Feel My Calories: Math that Even Mathematicians Can't Do Well

Recall the metabolic story of Jack and Jill from the previous section, "Inefficient Metabolism." You may have found yourself asking: if calories are what our cells use for energy, and this energy is what a homeostatic system regulates, then why didn't Jill feel fuller after eating 200 calories of food compared with inefficient Jack? Good question, because she most likely won't feel any fuller. While our cells can detect nutrients, our hunger and fullness is largely regulated by other factors not intrinsic to the nutrients we consume, at least in humans.

Among the most common nutrients manipulated in animal studies are proteins and carbohydrates, each of which has four calories per gram, and fats, which have nine calories per gram (making them a higher density load). In rats, foods containing the same total number of calories but differing in caloric density can significantly affect food intake.[1] For example, Robert Bolles and colleagues demonstrated greater preference in rats for a flavor associated with two grams of a four-calorie food than for a flavor associated with four grams of a two-calorie food.[2] Both foods had the same number of overall calories (eight), but the two-gram food was a more calorically dense load than the four-gram option. What they found was that rats receiving the higher density food preferred its flavor even when the calories were later removed. Thus, when given a choice between flavors associated with high- versus low-calorie dense foods, they consumed more of the flavor associated with the high calorie-dense food. In this study, the density of calories influenced what flavors rats liked or preferred to eat.

Humans, on the other hand, are not so savvy. It is no secret that most people love fatty foods, but explaining our tendency to consume high-fat foods in terms of their greater caloric density is not that simple. As mentioned previously, we tend to judge hunger and fullness more on learned factors not intrinsic to the nutritional value of the foods we consume. Yes, you will likely consume more of a high-fat food than a similar food that contains less fat, but if they are the same size and taste, you will likely feel just as full with fewer calories. In other words, to a large extent, when we eat, what we eat, and how much of it we eat is controlled by what we learn about food, not entirely by how many calories are in it. To illustrate this, let's look at how something seemingly as generic as the *visibility* and *convenience* of a high-fat food can influence consumption. Brian Wansink and his colleagues at the University of Illinois at Urbana-Champaign showed that increasing the visibility and convenience of chocolate increases consumption of that product.[3] In their study, the researchers placed thirty Hershey kisses in an uncovered container either on top of a desk (convenient and visible), in a desk drawer (convenient but not visible), or on a shelf far enough away that participants would have to get up from the desk to reach the chocolates (visible but not convenient). Efforts were made to ensure that all participants were equally hungry. The results showed that the more inconvenient the location of the chocolate, the less of it they ate—the group with the candies on the desk (convenient and visible) showed the greatest consumption of the chocolates. Thus, making the chocolates inconvenient reduced consumption of them and the calories associated with them, independent of hunger.

One application from this research would be to suggest making healthier food options more visible and convenient, especially for children. However, the application of this research is mostly to high-fat, high-sugar foods. Pay attention next time you use the checkout line at your local supermarket. What foods are convenient and visible as you wait for your groceries to be checked out? Do you find any lettuce or carrots? No, but there are Gobstoppers, Nerds, Hershey's Kisses for Valentine's Day, Milky Way and Snickers bars, Gummi Worms, and an assortment of chewing gums. Ironically, sometimes you will even find toothbrushes or dental floss by the cash register. What could be more convenient and accessible than the candy lining our checkout lanes? This is especially so for children, who are notoriously impulsive shoppers and remarkably effective negotiators with parents waiting to check out. Do you think the makers of these candies are unaware of this research, or do you think they use this kind of research as part of their marketing strategy? Of course they are aware! That is why candy is readily available in a place you must pass if you plan to obtain your food legally. I don't mean to imply that placing healthier foods at checkout aisles would guarantee we eat more of them, but Wansink and his colleagues have suggested as much—that increasing the availability and convenience of healthier food options such as fruits and vegetables could increase consumption of them as well. In this study, subjects did not start (or stop) eating the candies because they were hungry (or full). Instead, how much they ate depended on factors besides the calories—convenience and visibility. Yes, our cells can detect the calories we consume,[4] but we keep eating (or stop eating) despite this.

Take for another example the portion sizes of our meals. Wansink and his colleagues showed that increasing the size of a bucket of popcorn at the movies increased consumption of the popcorn, even when the popcorn was stale.[5] In fact, we are more likely to buy a larger portion of one food than to buy the same amount in two smaller portions. When McDonald's learned of this, its operators devised a novel method of increasing profits by asking the tempting question, "Would you like that supersized?" Even if you had no intention of supersizing your meal, you probably would if they asked, and most people have no trouble finishing this larger portion—they simply can't resist all those cheap calories. After all, at what point does anyone count the calories associated with supersizing when he or she is using the drive-through? Even if it were possible, most people will never count those calories, just the money they are supposedly saving. In essence, when it comes to counting calories, most people—yes, even mathematicians—can't count very well.

Regulating Long-Term Body Weight

Cellular metabolism regulates our daily short-term energy intake (most calories are expended or stored within an hour of a meal, and most researchers agree that a separate mechanism regulates long-term body weight. Thus it is no coincidence that, other things being equal, a person's body weight today is about the same as it was yesterday, and a week ago. For some reason, body weight remains fairly constant over a time period much longer than that between meals. It is most likely that the body is actively doing something to stabilize long-term weight, and this has important implications for what we must do to lose weight and keep it off. To understand how this works, we must understand the basics of how the body signals short-term hunger and satiety.

Short-term hunger signals. There are two known ways the body can signal hunger to the brain. The first is referred to as *glucoprivation*—a decline in the glucose available to cells, which causes hunger. The second is *lipoprivation*—a decline in fatty acids, i.e., fats or lipids available to cells, which also causes hunger. Receptors that detect these hunger signals are located in the liver (lipoprivation and glucoprivation detection) and the brain (glucoprivation detection). Animal research indicates that depriving the liver of the ability to metabolize (utilize for energy) either glucose (glucoprivation) or fatty acids (lipoprivation) causes hunger.[6] Compensation for lipoprivation requires increased intake of lipids; increased intake of glucose is ineffective at terminating these hunger signals. Similarly, compensation for glucoprivation requires increased intake of glucose; increased intake of lipids is ineffective at terminating these signals. Receptors in the brain, on the other hand, monitor levels of glucose only on the brain side of the blood-brain barrier—a semi-permeable barrier in which cells lining the capillary walls tighten so as to prevent water-soluble molecules from freely entering the brain. Recall that during the fasting phase of metabolism, the brain uses primarily glucose as energy. Thus its detectors are primarily sensitive to glucoprivation.

So how do our cells detect the availability of energy? Receptors on cells are sensitive to their own internal metabolic rate, instead of directly monitoring the availability of nutrients in the bloodstream.[7] Consider that energy in the blood is nothing more than unused energy—it is the money in our wallets. It doesn't make much sense to monitor this since it is more important that this energy is being used. It is like giving you a million dollars that you can't spend; you have plenty of money, but your short-term needs are not being met. Likewise, if our bodies have significant amounts of energy in the blood but none of it is being used, then we do not have useful energy. Thus, by monitoring internal metabolic rate (or the rate of energy use), where slower rates indicate less energy available in the blood, our cells are able to directly monitor the energy they actually use and indirectly monitor energy levels in the bloodstream. It is quite an efficient process for monitoring cellular metabolism and initiating hunger.

Short-term satiety signals. Signals relating to glucose and lipids precede a meal, but what factors contribute to ending the meal? Short-term satiety signals are an immediate consequence of eating, and include learned and biological factors. As food progresses toward absorption in the body, satiety signals are constantly being released (referred to as *anticipatory satiety*). Since it takes about an hour for the cells in our body to start receiving energy from the food we consume, it is important that we stop eating *before* our cells receive this energy. Without anticipatory satiety, we would consume too many calories in each meal. Thus, to limit overeating—finally a mechanism to help us not overeat—our digestive system sends satiety signals to the brain well before the cells receive the energy we consume. This is important, since (in theory) a homeostatic system shouldn't stop a signal to correct a problem until that problem has been corrected. In the case of feeding, though, our bodies stop the signal to eat well before this problem (signaled by low internal metabolic rate) has been corrected. This is yet another example of how a homeostatic system fails to fully account for feeding.

As food passes through the stomach, receptors monitor the energy consumed. Animal studies have shown that rats will adjust their subsequent meals when food is withdrawn from their stomachs.[8] This adjustment of subsequent meals is specific to the nutrient levels of foods, not the volume, since rats still compensate for nutritional losses following injections of a non-nutritious saline solution.[9] Those injections keep volume intake constant but reduce nutritional intake. The intestines also contain receptors that are sensitive to glucose, amino acids, and fatty acids. As food passes via the pylorus (a region at the junction of the stomach and duodenum) and duodenum (about the first ten inches of the intestines), satiety signals are sent to the brain.

So what are these signals and how do they reach the brain? Many hormones in the body appear to transmit satiety signals to the brain, including bombesin, leptin, and cholecystokinin (CCK). One primary satiety signal (one that is best understood) comes from the hormone referred to as CCK.[10] This hormone temporarily suppresses eating and is increasingly released as the entry of food to the duodenum increases. CCK also regulates the rate of stomach emptying, and therefore the rate at which the body receives energy. CCK can't cross the blood-brain barrier, so it can't enter the brain. Thus, it acts peripherally to reduce eating by activating a rich collection of CCK receptors located in the pylorus. These receptors then send messages to the brain. Ultimately these messages are received by a discrete region of the brain called the hypothalamus via the gastric branch of the vagus nerve—a branch of one of twelve cranial nerves extending to discrete brain structures. These twelve nerves are the only way (other than passing through the blood-brain barrier) to get chemical information to the brain. This signal allows the digestive system to provide feedback to the brain. Essentially, CCK keeps the brain informed constantly of what is going on in the intestines and allows the brain to respond accordingly by causing a sense of fullness.

Long-term regulation of short-term signals. So what does this have to do with long-term regulation of body weight? Well, we know that body weight is a determinant of food intake and that overall body weight appears to be regulated. For example, force-feeding studies in animals have shown that food intake falls as body weight increases;[11] starvation studies have shown that food intake increases as body weight falls.[12] This means that if you gain a lot of pounds, you are likely to reduce eating and return to your normal body weight. Likewise, if you lose a lot of weight, you are likely to eat more and return to your normal body weight. This is rather depressing for anyone looking to lose weight because it suggests that no matter what you do, your body will maintain the weight you want to avoid. The *set-point theory* for long-term body weight regulation has gained favor among many researchers in explaining how the body does this.

This theory posits that the body actively adjusts our sensitivity to foods and cues associated with foods so as to ensure that we maintain a constant body weight over time. It does this by adjusting how sensitive the brain is to satiety (and possibly hunger) signals. For example, CCK is less effective (i.e., more CCK is needed) at stopping eating when body weight has been reduced below normal levels. The system is designed to tempt you to eat more by preventing you from feeling as full as you otherwise would be. The result is increased food intake in the form of larger meals, not a larger number of meals.

Another way we regulate long-term body weight is to adjust the rate at which our cells use energy. If we increase the rate of cellular metabolism then we will reach satiety faster, and our meal sizes will be smaller. If we decrease the rate of cellular metabolism then it will take longer to reach satiety, and our meal sizes will be larger. Either strategy would be effective either to get us to gain weight (decreasing cellular metabolism) or lose weight (increasing cellular metabolism). Thus, when people diet to lose weight, their bodies immediately start getting them to gain it back either by decreasing their sensitivity to satiety hormones or by adjusting the rate at which their cells use energy. So, is there a loophole—a way around this? Theoretically there is, but unfortunately it means you have to be a patient weight loser.

Many researchers believe that the body is willing essentially to compromise "normal" body weight if we will lose the weight slowly (about one to two pounds per week at most). For example, (say) you weigh 150 pounds and you want to lose ten pounds. If you lose all ten pounds in a week, your body won't adjust to your new weight and will begin trying to make you eat more. But many researchers believe that if you lose the ten pounds over a ten-week period (one pound per week), your long-term body weight will adjust. By losing weight slowly, you allow the body to adjust its set point. You will have trained your body to regulate that lower weight, which has now become the "normal" weight your body will try to maintain. As will be evident by the end of this book, if you want to lose weight and eat healthier long-term, you must train your body to do so. This often takes time, although not more than a few weeks in most cases.

Notes

1. Booth, D.A. (1981). Hunger and satiety as conditioned reflexes. In Weiner, H., Hofer. M. A., & Stunkard, A. J. (Eds.), *Brain, Behavior, and Bodily Disease* (pp. 143-163). New York: Raven Press.
2. Bolles, R. C., Hayward, L., & Crandell, C. (1981). Conditioned taste preferences based on caloric density. *Journal of Experimental Psychology: Animal Behavior Processes, 7*, 59-69.
3. Painter, J. E., Wansink, B., & Hieggelke, J. B. (2002). How visibility and convenience influence candy consumption. *Appetite, 38*, 237-38.
4. Ritter, R. C., Brenner, L., & Yox, D. P. (1992). Participation of vagal sensory neurons in putative satiety signals from the upper gastrointestinal tract. In Ritter, S.,

Ritter, R. C., & Barnes, C. D. (Eds.), *Neuroanatomy and Physiology of Abdominal Vagal Afferents* (pp. 221-249). Boca Raton, Florida: CRC Press.

5. Wansink, B., & Kim, J. (2005). Bad popcorn in big buckets: Portion size can influence intake as much as taste. *Journal of Nutrition Education and Behavior, 37* (3), 242-245.

6. Friedman, M. I., Tordoff, M. G., & Ramirez, I. (1986). Integrated metabolic control of food intake. *Brain Research Bulletin, 17*, 855-859.

7. Nicolaidis, S. (1987). What determines food intake? The ischymetric theory. *News in Physiological Sciences, 2*, 104-107.

8. Davis, J. D., & Campbell, C. S. (1973). Peripheral control of meal size in the rat: Effect of sham feeding on meal size and drinking rate. *Journal of Comparative and Physiological Psychology, 83*, 379-387.

9. Deutsch, J. A., & Gonzalez, M. F. (1980). Gastric nutrient content signals satiety. *Behavioral and Neural Biology, 30*, 113-116.

10. Gibbs, J., Young, R. C., & Smith, G. P. (1973). Cholecystokinin decreases food intake in rats. *Journal of Comparative and Physiological Psychology, 84*, 488-495.

11. Wilson, F. A. W., OScalaidhe, S. P., & Goldman-Rakic, P. S. (1990). Identification of candidate genes for a factor regulating body weight in primates. *American Journal of Physiology, 259*, R1148-R1155.

12. Cabanac, M., & LaFrance, L. (1991). Facial consummatory responses in rats support the ponderostat hypothesis. *Physiology and Behavior, 50*, 179-183.

Chapter 3: Learning About Hunger and Fullness

All other things being equal, the larger our previous meal, the longer will be the interval until our next meal. This is partly (maybe largely) because we consume more calories in a larger meal, meaning it will take longer before we feel the need to eat again. Also, other things being equal, the longer the interval until the next meal, the more we will eat in that meal. A longer fast between meals would be associated with a greater need for calories at the next meal, which would explain why we eat more—but this is not entirely true. The fact is that we would eat again soon after a meal if we simply couldn't remember when (or how much) we ate last—and there is evidence to support this.

Consider a fascinating study conducted by Paul Rozin and colleagues.[1] This research group studied two amnesic patients who had almost no explicit memory for events that had occurred only minutes before. In particular, these patients had no recall of what foods they had just eaten. If calories were primary in regulating meal size and the intervals between meals, then simply knowing whether or not you had just eaten should have little bearing on feeding. Instead, on three occasions during the study, both patients willingly consumed a second meal when offered within thirty minutes after completion of the first meal, and they on several occasions began to consume a third meal when offered thirty minutes after completion of the second. Each meal contained upward of 700 calories. Since these patients had no recollection of whether or not they had eaten, let alone how much, they continued to eat. It is a rather compelling example of just how inept humans are at "feeling" their calories and how dependent people are on learned factors.

Calories are indubitably regulated, monitored, stored, and used by the body. It is also evident that at some level our bodies (specifically, the cells in our bodies) are aware of how many calories we consume. Unfortunately, our bodies are not good at sharing that information with our conscious selves. Humans tend to be very bad at estimating how many calories they consume. Even worse, we don't seem to completely experience hunger and fullness based on the number of calories we consume. Indeed, distractions while we eat will increase how many calories we consume. A recent study reported by Reuters news agency found that people eat an average of 44 percent more chips while watching the Late Show With David Letterman and 42 percent more while viewing the Tonight Show With Jay Leno than when they are not watching TV.[2] The more entertaining the program, the more people eat. This is not to say that we won't stop eating after we consume a large number of calories. We will stop eating, but not entirely because of the calories.

To illustrate this, Kissileff and colleagues conducted a series of experiments in which they offered subjects either soup (tomato and chicken noodle) or a combination of foods (cheese, crackers, jelly, and juice) as preload foods, with both choices being of equal caloric content, and then offered these same subjects a lunch (macaroni and beef casserole with tomatoes).[3] They were interested in knowing whether participants would eat the same number of calories in the lunch after consuming these isocaloric (equal in calories) preload foods. If they judge hunger and fullness based solely on how many calories they consume, then the participants should consume similar amounts of lunch on average after this preload. Instead, the experiments demonstrated that a preload of soup was more satiating than a preload of the combination of foods. Participants ate much less lunch if they consumed soup prior to lunch as opposed to the combination. Also, the total caloric intake (preload plus meal) was least when soup was the preload.

Explanations for this series of experiments have varied, but one intriguing explanation came from Barbara Rolls and colleagues, who raised the possibility that the perception of the foods we eat may contribute to hunger and fullness.[4] How full we feel after eating a food may be due very much to what we *think* we should feel after eating it. This means that we judge fullness and hunger on things we learn and not as much on things that our body regulates automatically (such as calories we consume). But why would one food make participants feel fuller than another of equal calories? In this chapter we will begin by answering this question and continue to review the many additional factors and beliefs that can affect how much we eat—ultimately affecting how many calories we consume. Once we understand what makes us feel full (other than calories), we can begin to develop simple strategies for feeling fuller longer on fewer calories.

A Calorie Is Not Just a Calorie: Snacking

Bellisle and colleagues recently measured the relative contributions of meals and snacks to daily food intake by using daily diaries in which participants recorded what they ate and drank for a few weeks.[5] They found that snacking between meals did not affect the amount consumed in a subsequent meal. They also reported that foods consumed as part of a meal were eaten in larger amounts than when they were consumed as snacks. No matter how many snacks participants ate, they still ate large meals, and they always ate their largest portions during meals. The macronutrient content and energy density of snack foods also do not appear to suppress subsequent intake during meals. For example,

Marmonier and colleagues gave subjects a high-fat (58% of energy from fat), a high-protein (77% of energy from protein), or a high-carbohydrate (84% of energy from carbohydrates) snack prior to dinner.[6] They found that snack composition had no effect on subsequent energy or macronutrient intake during dinner. No matter how many calories participants snacked on, snacking didn't decrease the size—and number of calories—of the subsequent meal.

Meals are generally eaten at specific times that vary by culture, and they are the highest caloric loads taken in at one time during the day.[7] Snacks, on the other hand, are eaten in smaller amounts and account for much fewer calories than meals. Still, it should be expected that the calories we consume while snacking to "hold us off" should have some effect on the size of subsequent meals. In fact, they have no apparent effect on how much we eat later. My colleagues and I recently showed that participants eat significantly more calories in a lunch after eating 500 kilocalories (k/cal) of "snack foods" than eating the same amount of "meal foods" before the lunch.[8] In this study, the snack and meal foods were the same—the only difference was whether subjects *thought* of them as snack or meal foods. The researchers noted that snack foods are rarely consumed to satiation. Most people do not fill up on snacks; they simple eat snacks to hold them over until the next meal. It is during the meal that most people eat until they feel full. This suggests that we learn snacks are not filling, and therefore we can eat more of them without feeling full; whereas, we learn meals *are* filling, which may be why eating what they consider to be meal foods before the lunch actually decreased the amount of food that participants ate during the lunch.

Also, based on this work it could reasonably be argued that cheese and crackers in the Kissileff and colleagues study were snack foods, and that people had a history of eating them as such and not becoming particularly full. Fruits are consumed as snacks or even as desserts but are not characteristically meal foods. Soup, on the other hand, is often consumed as a meal. It would therefore be sensed as more filling than the combination of the snack foods used in the Kissileff and colleagues 1984 experiments. While issues such as meal frequency or prolonging satiety have not been adequately addressed, these studies do support the preliminary suggestion that snacking between meals is ineffective in curbing appetite.

This research leads to two suggestions: First, a better approach to hunger between meals may be to *consume more meals of less quantity*. A person would feel fuller longer by eating a small meal between lunch and dinner than if he or she ate the same amount of calories in a snack. Second, if you absolutely need your snacks, then you could *begin eating snack foods as part of your meal*. In theory, by eating these foods as part of a meal, they would become associated with the sensation of fullness—this would allow you to feel fuller sooner when consuming these snack foods later. Still, at present this suggestion is speculative and more research is needed to determine if this is a likely result.

A Calorie Is Not Just a Calorie: Drinking

Some researchers would have you believe that a calorie is just a calorie, no matter where it comes from.[9] While this may be true for how we use calories, it is not accurate at all for how we "sense" them, especially when we drink them. For example, consumption of energy-containing beverages is associated with an increase in energy intake and obesity. Studies conducted in children and adolescents have shown that consumption of sugar-sweetened drinks was associated with increased energy intake and risk of obesity.[10,11] When adults are provided with sweetened drinks to consume as desired, those given caloric drinks show significantly greater energy intake and body weight after several weeks than those provided with noncaloric drinks.[12] Unfortunately, these sweetened beverages (such as soda) provide few nutrients other than calories and don't appear to change how many calories we eat.

Alternatively, some reports cite evidence that various beverages differ in their effects on satiety and food intake. Specifically, these studies show that the addition of protein, fat, or fiber (nutrients commonly found in the foods we eat) to a beverage enhances satiety[13]; therefore, we stop eating earlier in a meal to compensate for the calories we consume in the beverage. This study showed that satiety is greater after consumption of a liquid meal replacement containing a mix of sugar, fat, and protein, compared with an isocaloric beverage containing only sugar. Other studies have shown that energy-dense, milk-based drinks reduce intake—and therefore caloric intake—at a subsequent meal.[14]

Still, it is impractical to consider that the human population is going to begin drinking its energy in the years to come. Also, many of these studies tested whether caloric beverages consumed *before* a meal would affect energy intake. As we reviewed in the previous section, even the solid foods we eat or snack on (as opposed to liquid drinks) before a meal will have little effect on energy intake during a meal; i.e., we will still consume a "full" meal. Rolls and colleagues recently tested whether total energy intake at a meal is influenced by the energy and nutrient content of beverages we consume *during* a meal. Their research shows that when caloric beverages are consumed with a meal they add to energy intake from food, without significantly affecting ratings of satiety.[15] In other words, participants did not feel fuller sooner in the meal and they failed to compensate for the energy they were drinking by eating less.

There is a great deal of convincing evidence that we will not compensate for the calories we drink by reducing the calories we eat.[16,17] Thus, while people generally are bad at counting the calories they eat, they are even worse at counting the calories they drink. Unfortunately, caffeine is an addictive drug contained in many caloric beverages such as soda and coffee. Giving up soda (or coffee) completely may be unrealistic for some, although even cutting back on caloric drinks (especially sodas, sweetened teas, lemonades, etc.) can result in large weight losses. For example, top dieticians from the American Dietetic Association[18] report that a person can lose up to twenty-five pounds in a year simply by eliminating a twenty-ounce bottle of Coca-Cola every day and consuming Diet Coke instead. For those beverages that don't contain caffeine, the change should be even easier. Instead of whole milk, for example, switch to one percent—if your milk consumption is eight ounces a day, dietitians say you'll lose five pounds in a year.

As it turns out, though, switching to foods that are not part of a person's standard diet is difficult to do in the long run. While we can't feel our calories, we do learn to like them, and we eat what we like. It is so often overlooked that switching any aspect of your diet is not easy to do long-term. Many people have good intentions initially to stay on a diet, but staying on most diets long-term is easier said than done. Few, if any, experts would say otherwise. Ultimately the key to feeling fuller longer on fewer calories is to start eating the calories that make you feel full—and we don't feel full on the calories we drink. The bottom line: simply reducing or eliminating the calories you drink from your diet will result in fewer calories consumed (and likely weight loss) without leaving you feeling hungry.

Sensory-Specific Satiety

Fullness is undoubtedly a physiological phenomenon; but, as mentioned, calories are not the most influential cause of fullness. Other, learned factors can cause the physiological changes necessary to produce satiety and fullness. To understand these learned factors that cause fullness, it is important to distinguish between liking and wanting. Do we stop eating a meal because we stop liking it, or because we stop wanting it, or both? This question has turned out to be more difficult than anticipated. For example, liking or rating of pleasantness for a food does not decline with consumption.[19] Our *wanting* to consume a food declines, but the taste of the food is still rated as pleasant or *liked*. However, subsequent studies have shown strong correlation between a person's liking and wanting for foods served in a meal. These findings suggest that as we stop *wanting* a specific food, we stop *liking* it as well. Landmark studies by Barbara Rolls and colleagues have made some sense of these apparent contradictions in liking versus wanting.

These researchers initially considered whether foods become less pleasurable as we become fuller. After all, since we specifically choose foods we take pleasure in eating, it seems logical that fullness could be linked with pleasure or liking. As it turns out, while few people self-report that they stop eating because the foods in general stop tasting good, they also report decreases in liking for specific foods in a meal—termed *sensory-specific satiety*.[20] If people are asked why they stopped eating at the end of a large two-course meal, they most often report that they terminated the meal because of fullness. But if they are asked why they stopped eating specific foods at the end of each course, they are most likely to report that they are simply tired of eating those foods.[21] In other words, specific foods in the meal become less pleasurable to eat.

Sensory-specific satiety occurs when a food consumed within a meal is reported as less pleasant and the person does not want to have any more of it. This is probably something our ancestors knew a long time ago. Very few cultures (if any) eat just one food in a traditional meal. A meal is characterized in almost all cultures by multiple foods, courses, and servings. There are appetizers, main meals, and desserts. We don't eat only turkey for Thanksgiving. We eat stuffing, cranberry sauce, corn, gravy, and other foods during the feast. Then there is the dessert: a variety of pies, ice creams, and pastries that will make most any full stomach stretch a little more. Almost by definition, a meal must include courses or a selection of foods. As we eat at the table we ask, "Will you pass the potatoes?" or, "May I have another helping of dessert?" Meals offer variety, maybe because this ensures we will eat more—again, before the famine our bodies are conditioned to expect but which is not likely to come in Western society. Maybe our ancestors knew that we get full too fast on just one food, so they established the tradition of the "meal" to increase variety and therefore consumption before we experience fullness.

Recently, Barbara Rolls and her colleagues gathered evidence indicating how we judge fullness in regard to specific foods. They tested whether the change in rating of pleasantness after consuming a food is related either to the volume (amount of food consumed) or to the energy content of the food.[22] On each of three days, thirty-six women consumed one of three milk-based liquid foods that varied in energy content and volume, but were matched for palatability and macronutrient composition. Participants rated the pleasantness of the liquid foods and four other foods both immediately before and after consuming the liquid food. This study showed that doubling the volume of the liquid food that was consumed, without changing the energy content, significantly decreased pleasantness ratings of the liquid food and increased sensory-specific satiety. In other words, how "tired" we are of eating a food depends on how much we have eaten (volume), not on how many calories we consumed (nutrients). These findings could also explain why soup was more satiating than the combination of cheese, crackers, jelly, and juice in the 1984 Kissileff et al. experiments—the soup in that test was a greater volume load than the combination, which would explain why it was more filling.

This research has two important implications for learning how to feel fuller on fewer calories. First, *we eat less with less variety* in a single meal. Simply limiting the variety of foods you eat in a meal will allow you to feel fuller sooner; i.e., you will consume fewer calories before feeling satiated. Still, this suggestion comes with an important caveat: variety is considered good for health. Therefore, strategies for feeling fuller with fewer calories must limit variety *within a meal*, without limiting the variety of foods we eat in our diets overall. To do this, a dieter might consider eating less variety within a meal— say, two food options instead of three or four—and also increase variety from meal to meal—say, eat a different food at breakfast, lunch, and dinner each day or week, so that the overall variety of your diet keeps you healthy, but feeling fuller longer with fewer calories.

Second, we judge fullness on *how much we eat*. This means that we will feel just as full after eating a slice of high-calorie dessert as we would eating the same amount with fewer calories. One solution would be to eat lower-caloric foods (such as vegetables and salads) earlier in a meal. This way you will presumably fill up before you get to the higher-calorie foods. In fact, an entire dieting regiment referred to as "volumetrics" (authored by Barbara Rolls) is largely based on this suggestion[23]—because it is simple and practical. Still, this also comes with a caveat: calories are associated with how we learn to like foods (we learn to like calorie-dense foods). What this means is that decreasing the calories will not change how full you feel, but it could affect how much you like these foods—this is discussed in detail in chapter 8.

Food Selection, Preferences, and Energy Density

As a child, did you ever think you were ripped off because your brother or sister received more presents than you did, even though the total value that each sibling received was the same? If you are a parent, maybe you have experienced the stress of trying to explain this to a child who was convinced you loved the other child more because you bought him or her more presents. Interestingly, conventional dieting wisdom suggests that we treat food the same way. In other words, we tend to assume that we consume more calories with more pieces of food even when the calories of the foods were actually the same. This turns out to be false wisdom (at least empirically).

Although some reports suggest that reducing bite size does decrease the amount we eat, these reports have been difficult to replicate, suggesting that factors other than bite size are causing differences in eating. A study by Spiegel and colleagues varied bite size of sandwiches and measured rate of consumption and total amount consumed.[24] They found that rate of intake was higher for foods larger in bite size, but total amount consumed was constant across conditions. Conventional dieting advice is to cut food into smaller pieces so that it looks like more food, but recent reports contradict this suggestion.[25] For example, while we chew larger portions of food more efficiently (grams ingested per chew) and ingest these foods faster (grams ingested per minute), this has little impact on how much we consume in the overall meal. Cutting foods into smaller pieces does not reduce the amount of food you will eat—you don't get fuller faster, you simply eat slower. In fact, it is most common for researchers to observe meal size decline as a result of smaller bites only when the variety of foods offered is limited.[26] This finding (as reviewed in the previous section) may be more attributed to sensory-specific satiety cues than to the size of the bites, since only a few foods were offered (sometimes only one food).

On the other hand, in studies involving buffets where subjects are allowed to consume a variety of courses (including desserts) in any order they wish, three closely related factors appear to have greatest influence over satiety: food selection, preferences, and energy density. The pattern of eating buffet-style meals indicates that obese men (compared with lean men) select more-palatable (or preferred) foods early in the meal—foods that tend to contain more calories per gram than the other foods. Since we judge fullness based on how much we eat (more so than how many calories we eat), obese men end up eating similar amounts of food overall, but gram for gram they consume significantly more calories than lean men. The main implication of this research focuses on the knowledge that obesity is associated with selection of more-preferred foods that contain a lot of calories. Pies, pastries, and cakes are not only sweet, but also contain lots of calories. Hamburgers and steaks are not only high in fat, but also contain lots of calories. We put salt on French fries but, of course, they also contain lots of calories. The fact is that the foods we prefer tend to be high in calories, and if we eat them first in a meal (or if they are all that we eat for our meal) then we end up consuming a lot of calories without overeating per se. We will essentially feel full when we have eaten enough.

Thus, by eating more calories earlier in a meal, we ensure that our meals will be rich with calories before we ever experience fullness from the amount of food we have eaten. Therefore, eating calorie-depleted foods (such as highly nutritious but low-calorie fruits and vegetables) earlier in a meal may actually help us consume fewer calories prior to feeling full. This suggestion comes with an important caveat: We like high-calorie foods; therefore, eliminating them (or even significantly reducing them) from our diets is difficult, even unrealistic for long-term success. Strategies to increase liking for flavors associated with lower-calorie foods will be discussed at greater length in chapter 8.

Portion Size

While bite size has little effect on how much we consume, portion size has a considerable effect. There is a plethora of evidence suggesting that as the portion size of a meal is increased, so also is energy consumption.[27] Studies have shown that doubling the portion size of foods leads to an 18% to 25% increase in consumption for foods typically eaten in a meal (such as spaghetti) and a 30% to 45% increase for foods typically eaten as snacks.[28] Many children may have been conditioned to eat this way. Parents commonly tell children, "Eat what's on your plate!" with little regard for a child's hunger or satiety. Children tend to be reinforced for eating everything that is in front of them, and punished for not doing so. In other words, children are punished because they stop eating when they are full! Thus, children learn to judge fullness and hunger based on portion or meal sizes, not on their own feelings of hunger and satiety.[29]

Portion size appears to affect eating in three important ways. First, portion size is not correlated with ratings of hunger and fullness.[30] Even when portion size is doubled, subjects still report similar ratings of hunger and fullness after the meal. This finding appears to be specific to a meal, though. Larger portion sizes of snacks are associated instead with lower ratings of hunger. Still, this effect of greater satiety is rather short-term since (as previously described) snacks have no effect on the amount consumed in a meal served only minutes later. Also, the weight of food (closely associated with portion size) can affect satiety[31]—the heavier a food portion, the fuller a person feels. This may explain why snack foods, which tend to be light (chips, popcorn, pretzels, etc.), do not significantly affect the size of a subsequent meal. Regardless, increased portion sizes and heavier portions will increase overall caloric intake over the course of days.

Second, it is difficult for humans to distinguish between portion sizes.[32] When portion size is doubled, a subject will consume the entire portion. Even when subjects are able to distinguish between portion sizes, they will still consume larger amounts of food when given larger portion sizes. Thus energy intake increases with larger portion sizes, even when we are aware that the portion size is larger than normal—this is the supposed genius behind supersizing. If the food is in front of us, we apparently will eat all of it, or at least we'll try.

Third, as portion size increases, post-meal rating of the taste of the food decreases. After-meal ratings of liking are lower following consumption of greater amounts (weight or volume) of a solid food compared with the consumption of smaller amounts of the same food in a meal. Still, this doesn't seem to change how portion size affects eating behavior. For example, even when the food we eat presumably tastes bad (such as stale popcorn), we will still eat more if we are given larger portions.[33]

While the mechanisms that cause us to make judgments of fullness, hunger, and pleasantness based on portion sizes are not well known, this research still has potentially important implications for successful dieting. The obvious implication is to *decrease the portions of high-calorie foods,* and even to compensate for this by increasing portions of healthier foods. This would allow you to consume similar amounts of food in your diet, but with fewer net calories. Of course, the most successful way to diet long-term would be to learn to *like* low-calorie foods and *eat less* of high-calorie foods—again, such strategies are discussed at length in chapter 8.

Making Sense of Hunger and Fullness

The human population in general has developed a wide range of simple and complex social cues necessary for all aspects of survival, including food, sex, social inclusion, etc. Food has been at the center of our social interaction. It is such a socially triggered phenomenon that we tend to eat more just because we are in the company of others.[34] Children who come home with good report cards get pizza or ice cream; businessmen close multimillion-dollar deals while dining at expensive restaurants; a boy takes a girl he likes out to dinner to impress her; a bride and groom celebrate their vows at a reception rich with appetizers, main dishes, and desserts; and families celebrate most any important holiday (secular or sacred) with a feast. We even eat for no good reason, as comedian Jim Carrey popularized in the movie, *The Grinch Who Stole Christmas*: "Am I eating cause I'm bored?"

Food has a part in almost every aspect of human culture and tradition. It should, therefore, not be surprising that we have developed such an intricate set of cognitive rules for hunger and satiety—rules that include which foods we consume and how much food is offered. In human culture, hunger is not the only reason to eat. When, where, how, with whom, and why you eat vary with the occasion and the season. Thus it makes intuitive sense that we would develop strategies for determining hunger and fullness that are not intrinsic to the calories we consume; we do not eat simply because we need calories. This leads to some practical advice for parents: allow children to feed on an "on demand" schedule—let your children control when and how much they eat.[35] By allowing infants control over the timing of meals (when to eat) and meal size (the amount eaten), parents can teach their children to be sensitive to internal biological cues for hunger and satiety. All evidence indicates that children can regulate their energy intake this way. By six months of age, infants who are fed "on demand" will begin—on their initiative—eating their largest meals at night prior to sleep—which is their longest fast between meals.[36]

The learned components of hunger and satiety come with important benefits for those wanting to change their diets long-term. Most of our judgments concerning hunger and fullness are *learned* (not innately associated with the calories we consume). Since we can feel hungry or full independent of our caloric needs, we can learn how to feel fuller without consuming all those calories. Still, lower consumption of calories in a diet is associated with lower preference for that diet, and most preferences are learned as well. This means that we can learn to like eating fewer calories as well as feel fuller after eating lower-calorie meals! But before we move into this, the next section will review briefly why dieters seem always to revert to their preferred diets, thus (partly) answering the question: why is changing our diets so hard to do long-term? By understanding key factors that make us want and like our diets, we will be able to appreciate why dieting is a lot more than just hunger and fullness.

Notes

1. Rozin, P., Dow, S., Moscovitch, M., & Rajaram, S. (1998). What causes humans to begin and end a meal? A role for memory for what has been eaten, as evidenced by a study of multiple meal eating in amnesic patients. *Psychological Science*, 9 (5), 392-396.
2. Reported online by Reuters: "Entertaining TV programs make you eat, study finds," 3 June 2007.
3. Kissileff, H. R., Gruss, L. P., Thornton, J., & Jordan, H. A. (1984). The satiating efficiency of foods. *Physiology & Behavior, 32,* 319-332.
4. Rolls, B. J., Fedoroff, I. C., Guthrie, J. F., & Laster, L. J. (1990). Foods with different satiating effects in humans. *Appetite, 15,* 115-126.

5. Bellisle, F., Dalix, A. M., Mennen, L., Galan, P., Hercberg, S., de Castro, J. M., & Gausseres, N. (2003). Contribution of snacks and meals in the diet of French adults: A diet-diary study. *Physiology & Behavior*, 79 (2), 183-189.

6. Marmonier, C., Chapelot, D., & Louis-Sylvestre, J. (2000). Effects of macronutrient content and energy density of snacks consumed in a satiety state on the onset of the next meal. *Appetite*, 34 (2), 161-168.

7. de Castro, J. M., Brewer, E. M., Elmore, D. K., & Orozco, S. (1990). Social facilitation of the spontaneous meal size of humans occurs regardless of time, place, alcohol or snacks. *Appetite*, *15*, 80-101.

8. Capaldi, E. D., Owens, J. Q., & Privitera, G. J. (2006). Isocaloric meal and snack foods differentially affect eating behavior. *Appetite*, 46 (2), 117-123.

9. Heilbronn, L. K., de Jonge, L., Frisard, M. I., DeLany, J. P., et al. (2006). Effect of 6-month calorie restriction on biomarkers of longevity, metabolic adaptation, and oxidative stress in overweight individuals: a randomized controlled trial. *JAMA*, 295 (13), 1539-1548.

10. Berkey, C. S., Rockett, H. R. H., Field, A. E., Gillman, M. W., & Colditz, G. A. (2004). Sugar-added beverages and adolescent weight change. *Obesity Research, 12*, 778–788.

11. Ludwig, D. S., Peterson, K. E., & Gortmaker, S. L. (2001). Relation between consumption of sugar-sweetened drinks and childhood obesity: A prospective, observational analysis. *Lancet, 357*, 505–508.

12. Raben, A., Vasilarasm, T. H., Moller, A. C., & Astrup, A. (2002). Sucrose compared with artificial sweeteners: Different effects on ad libitum food intake and body weight after 10 wk of supplementation in overweight subjects. *American Journal of Clinical Nutrition, 76*, 721–729.

13. St-Onge, M-P. , Rubiano, F., Jones, A., Greenfield, D., Ferguson, P. W., Akrabawi, S., & Heymsfield, S. B. (2004). Added thermogenic and satiety effects of a mixed nutrient vs. a sugar-only beverage. *International Journal of Obesity, 28*, 248–253.

14. Rolls, B. J., Castellanos, V. H., Halford, J. C., Kilara, A., Panyam, D., Pelkman, C. L., Smith, G. P., & Thorwart, M. L. (1998). Volume of food consumed affects satiety in men. *American Journal of Clinical Nutrition, 67*, 1170–1177.

15. DellaValle, D. M., Roe, L. S., & Rolls, B. J. (2005). Does the consumption of caloric and non-caloric beverages with a meal affect energy intake? *Appetite, 44*, 187-193.

16. Almiron-Roig, E., Flores, S. Y., & Drewnowski, A. (2004). No difference in satiety or in subsequent energy intakes between a beverage and a solid food. *Physiology & Behavior*, 82 (4), 671-677.

17. Almiron-Roig, E., & Drewnowski, A. (2003). Hunger, thirst, and energy intakes following consumption of caloric beverages. *Physiology & Behavior*, 79 (4-5), 767-773.

18. Reported online by Prevention.com: "100 smartest diet tips ever," 4 Dec 2006.

19. Blundell, J. E., & Rogers, P. J. (1991). Hunger, hedonics, and the control of satiation and satiety. In M. Friedman, M. Tordoff, & M. Kare (Eds.), *Chemical senses, appetite, and nutrition* (vol. 4, pp. 127-148). New York: Marcel Dekker.

20. Rolls, B. J. (1986). Sensory-specific satiety. *Nutrition Reviews, 44*, 93-101.

21. Mook, D.G., & Votaw, M.C. (1992). How important is hedonism? Reasons given by college students for ending a meal. *Appetite, 18*, 69-75.

22. Bell, E. A., Roe, L. S., & Rolls, B. J. (2003). Sensory-specific satiety is affected more by volume than by energy content of a liquid food. *Physiology & Behavior*, 78 (4-5), 593-600.

23. Rolls, B. (2007). The Volumetrics Eating Plan: Techniques and Recipes for Feeling Full on Fewer Calories. New York: HarperCollins Publishers.

24. Spiegel, T. A., Kaplan, J. M., Tomassini, A., & Stellar, E. (1993). Bite size, ingestion rate, and meal size in lean and obese women. *Appetite*, 21 (2), 131-145.

25. Spiegel, T. A. (1999). Rate of intake, bites, and chews: The interpretation of lean-obese differences. *Neuroscience & Biobehavioral Reviews*, 24 (2), 229-237.

26. Yeomans, M.R., Gray, R.W., Mitchell, C.J., & True, S. (1997). Independent effects of palatability and within-meal pauses on intake and appetite ratings in human volunteers. *Appetite, 29*, 61-76.

27. Kral, T. V. E. (2006). Effects of hunger and satiety, perceived portion size and pleasantness of taste of varying portion size of foods: A brief review of selected studies. *Appetite, 46*, 103-105.

28. Fisher, J. O., Rolls, B. J., & Birch, L. L. (2001). Effects of repeated exposure of a large portion-sized entrée on children's eating. *Obesity Research, 9*, 76S.

29. Birch, L. L., McPhee, L., Shoba, B. C., Steinberg, L., & Krehbiel, R. (1987). Clean up your plate: Effects of child feeding practices on the conditioning of meal size. *Learning and Motivation, 18*, 301-317.

30. Kral, T. V. E., Roe, L. S., & Rolls, B. J. (2004). Combined effects of energy density and portion size on energy intake in women. *American Journal of Clinical Nutrition, 79*, 962–968.

31. de Graaf, C., & Hulshuf, T. (1996). Effects of weight and energy content of preloads on subsequent appetite and food intake. *Appetite, 26*, 139-151.

32. Kral, T. V. E., Meengs, J. S., Wall, D. E., Roe, L. S., & Rolls, B. J. (2003). Effect on food intake of increasing the portion size of all foods over two consecutive days. *The Federation of American Societies for Experimental Biology Journal, 17*, A809 (abstract).

33. Wansink, B., & Kim, J. (2005). Bad popcorn in big buckets: Portion size can influence intake as much as taste. *Journal of Nutrition Education and Behavior, 37* (3), 242-245.

34. de Castro, J.M. (1990). Social facilitation of duration and size but not rate of the spontaneous meal intake in humans. *Physiology & Behavior, 47*, 1129-1135.

35. Satter, E. (1990). The feeding relationship: Problems and interventions. *The Journal of Pediatrics, 117*, S181-S189.

36. Birch, L. L., & Fisher, J. A. (1996). The role of early experience in the development of children's eating behavior. In E. D. Capaldi (Ed.), *Why We Eat What We Eat: The Psychology of Eating* (pp. 113-141). Washington, D.C.: American Psychological Association.

SECTION II: Why Dieting Is So Difficult

Chapter 4: The Pleasure Centers

Over millennia, the human brain has evolved by adding new brain matter on top of old brain matter. From oldest to youngest (in the course of evolution), the brain can be divided generally into three sections: hindbrain, midbrain, and forebrain. The forebrain consists of the neocortex (or "new" cortex) and other structures involved in the advanced processing of environmental stimuli (anything we hear, see, smell, or feel). Its functions reflect the unique cognitive abilities of humans today, including more-advanced processing of sensory information (including taste and smell). This is why we are capable of so many cognitive strategies for feeling hungry and full. The midbrain, a region formed earlier in human history, controls more-rudimentary functions, such as the basic motivational and rewarding aspects of eating and sexual behaviors necessary for sustaining life and procreation. Still more-basic functions such as sneezing, coughing, vomiting, and breathing are regulated by hindbrain structures, which are considered the regions formed earliest in human history.

Each brain region is linked to the others, which allows our more-advanced "new" cortex to acquire higher processing of our more-rudimentary behaviors (such as eating and sex). Cell bodies (referred to as nuclei) in the older hindbrain and midbrain regions extend axons, or lines of communication, to cell bodies in the forebrain. You might think of cell bodies and axons as landline telephone receivers and telephone lines, respectively. Similar to how telephone lines extend from one receiver to another, axons extend from one cell body to another. In the same way that our voices (i.e., communication) are transmitted from one telephone receiver to another, neurotransmitters are "transmitted" from one cell body to another via axons. Ultimately, neurotransmitters provide information to cell bodies, which in turn use this information to influence behavior. Connecting the lines of communication via axons between our more-basic midbrain (and hindbrain) cell bodies and the newer forebrain cell bodies ensures more-advanced processing of motivationally relevant stimuli, including food rewards.

Connecting the Lines of Communication

The limbic system, a forebrain system often referred to as the *pleasure center* of the brain, is composed of a network of cell bodies and axons involved in learning, memory, emotion, and reinforcement. This system is considered a major pleasure center because the intense activation of limbic regions in the brain gives rise to a host of pleasurable eating and sexual responses. One structure in the limbic system known to be largely responsible for coding the reinforcement level of food rewards is the nucleus accumbens (NAcc). This brain structure (in addition to being part of the limbic system) receives input about rewarding stimuli from dopamine-producing neurons in the ventral tegmental area (VTA), which originates in the midbrain and extends axons to cell bodies in the limbic system and forebrain.[1] Dopamine is specifically produced by two midbrain structures: the VTA and the Substantia Nigra. While these two regions constitute very little of the surface area of the brain, they have a profound effect on behavior. Specifically, they not only affect how reinforcing we perceive food rewards to be, but also influence what foods we want and are motivated to consume.[2]

Cell bodies in a variety of brain regions responsible for learning and memory (hippocampus), emotion (amygdala), reinforcement (nucleus accumbens), and decision-making (prefrontal cortex) receive dopamine input from the VTA concerning biologically needed stimuli, including information about food and sex. In terms of food reward, dopamine (directly or indirectly) is the primary neurotransmitter responsible for causing the foods we like to be reinforcing. It informs the forebrain of stimuli we need (such as food) and enables behavioral responses to obtain it. In essence, the dopamine system is opportunistic: anything that stimulates its release is wanted, liked, and in many ways pursued without discrimination. The input of dopamine extends from the older midbrain (specifically in the VTA) to cell bodies in many regions of the newer forebrain. Again, since the three sections of our brain are interlinked, this allows the more-advanced processing of our newer forebrain to influence the more basic-functions of eating.

The Midbrain Dopamine System

The VTA influences behavior via its production of the chemical neurotransmitter dopamine. Neurotransmitters in the brain (including dopamine) are the chemical messengers that provide messages to neighboring neurons, which receive these messages (a *neuron* refers to a single cell body and axon). Dopamine is primarily involved in goal-directed behavior. It appears to be more important for the behavioral activation that secures the goal (or avoidance of aversive stimuli) than for mediation of the reward itself. The brain evolved this system of dopamine-producing neurons to respond to natural rewards, such as food—rewards necessary to survival. It is a matter of evolutionary survival and fitness that we consume safe and nutritious foods in order to reach a mature age in which to procreate. (Not surprisingly, this system of neurons also responds to sexual stimuli.)

Humans discovered how to stimulate this system artificially with drugs—all classes of drugs stimulate this same dopamine system.[3] Indeed, anyone who has gone through the struggle of drug addiction understands how powerful is the dopamine system in controlling motivated behavior. Yes, this means the midbrain dopamine response to cocaine, marijuana, heroin, nicotine, and other drugs is difficult to distinguish from the dopamine response to food rewards. The system was designed to make motivationally important behaviors very rewarding, since they are necessary for survival. Many researchers believe that when individuals become addicted to drugs, the drugs become as motivationally relevant as food is to the individual. This partly explains why addicts have such a difficult time quitting long-term. The dopamine response is requiring them to seek out drugs, since anything that can stimulate this midbrain dopamine is assumed to be needed for life, regardless of whether it truly is or not.

Rewards act at least as importantly as *hedonic incentives*—our motivation to consume liked foods. This causes neural representations that elicit motivation and goal pursuit, rather than mere habit. We don't simply seek out food; instead, we are actively seeking out foods that we *like*. This system complements physiological drive states primarily by increasing the perceived hedonic incentive value of the corresponding reward; e.g., food looks and tastes better when we are hungry. Thus, we don't simply eat; we eat for the *pleasure* of eating. In other words, we don't eat just any food; we mostly consume those foods we like. The dopamine system is largely responsible for this pattern of eating—it biases our culinary choices by actively informing our forebrain to seek out specifically the foods we like.

If we have a choice between a liked food and a not-so-liked food, we will often choose the liked food even when this is not necessarily the choice we want to make. Say, for example, you go out to eat with the intention of ordering healthy foods. As you read through the menu, I'm sure you'll come across many healthy food options—but often you will choose the less-healthy options that you prefer, even though this was not your original intention. Many people report that "it just looks too good to resist"—in part because the dopamine system is influencing the forebrain to choose these less-healthy but preferred menu options. Dopamine makes us *want* what we like, and it is very good at its job—sooner or later, you will submit to this midbrain dopamine system. That is one reason this book emphasizes that the *only* way to stay on a diet long-term is to learn to like or prefer the healthier food options, not just to start consuming them. Learning to *like* healthier food options will, in theory, allow these healthier foods to stimulate midbrain dopamine neurons, which will produce a *wanting* for the healthier foods as well. We eat what we like because the dopamine system *wants* what we like. Long-term dieting success is therefore partly dependent on appeasing this dopamine reward system.

Wanting Versus Liking

The dopamine response is thought to be responsible for increasing *wanting* independent of *liking*, and vice versa.[4] Dopamine-receiving neurons in the orbitofrontal cortex—a brain region located above our orbits (eye sockets)—have been shown to respond to the relative preference between food rewards.[5] For example, research with monkeys has demonstrated that when given a choice between a liked food and a more-preferred food (such as a raisin, which monkeys really like), neurons show preferentially stronger dopamine responses (higher rates of dopamine release between neurons, or "stronger communication") when the more-preferred food is presented, and monkeys subsequently show a behavioral preference for this food as well. Thus, the dopamine response itself appears to be involved in *incentive salience*—a wanting for more attractive or preferred food rewards.

Still, dopamine may also mediate important aspects of reward liking as well. Neurons in the orbitofrontal cortex also respond to the relative hedonic or liked qualities of foods. For example, neurons in this region will increase rates of activity when fatty foods are consumed. This is considered evidence that neurons are preferentially responding to fats. Considering that fat contains more calories per gram (nine) than any other nutrient we consume, it makes sense that we should like it. After all, it is the only nutrient our body can use between meals—that is, during the fasting phase of metabolism. Unfortunately, times have changed. The feast and famine world of our ancestors has been replaced with a feast and feast some more existence, where food availability is just another thing the average person (including me) takes for granted. Evolution is simply too slow to adjust, and therefore we continue to like those high-calorie fats for the famine that is supposed to follow the feast.

Dopamine is released during both appetitive (food seeking) and consummatory (food consumption) aspects of behavior. Thus, dopamine likely plays a role in both the motoric activation required to achieve a goal (e.g., wanting) and in the reward itself (e.g., liking). Distinctions between neural systems of *wanting* and *liking* rewards have emerged from studies of natural rewards (especially sweet-tasting rewards). In human infants, the sweet sucrose taste elicits a set of facial expressions of liking (tongue protrusion, smile, etc.), whereas the bitter taste of quinine elicits facial expressions of dislike (gape, etc). Opioid peptide neurotransmitters—which are often released in conjunction with dopamine—are released within the NAcc and are known to enhance food acceptance and increase liking for food rewards, such as sucrose.[6] The neurochemical dissociation between *liking* and *wanting* has important relevance to our diets. Similar to the addict who continues to want a drug that he or she would prefer not to use anymore, we are probably addicted to our foods—although the key distinction is that we need to consume food to sustain life. Still, we will consume foods that the dopamine system wants to consume, even if we would prefer to eliminate them from our diets. (The possibility of dietary addiction is discussed at greater length toward the end of chapter 5.) One of the few known ways to "beat" this system is to learn to like healthier food options as well, so that they will also stimulate the midbrain dopamine system largely responsible for making foods pleasurable. This, in theory, will allow dieters to *want* healthier food options that they have learned to *like* as part of a preferred diet.

Dopamine and Learning

Still, a shift of liking is a bit more complicated. Not only do food rewards cause an increase in dopamine, so also does *anything* associated with these food rewards. Whatever is associated with food rewards such as sweet, salt, and fat can cause dopamine over time to respond to those predictive cues and not to the food itself. In other words, our dopamine system is actively seeking out not only the food rewards, but also anything that can predict them.[7] Thus, we don't need to eat the cake; all we need is to see it, or smell it baking, and our dopamine levels will rise in anticipation of the dessert. This contributes to our need to consume diet-typical foods—not only do we like sweet-tasting, fatty foods, we also like anything that predicts them. So simply to stop eating these foods will not eliminate the midbrain dopamine response. Dopamine neurons arouse motivation to respond to whatever stimulus is appropriate at the moment, leading to permanent changes in the structure of neurons in the brain. This means we learn about more than just the foods we eat; we learn about everything in the environment that predicts the possibility of eating them.

An *associative hypothesis* suggests that we learn to predict or expect the occurrence of food rewards. Dopamine responds with phasic (sudden) activations at the time rewards are presented and with phasic depressions at the time an otherwise expected reward is omitted. This depression is hypothesized to be a prediction error signal and implies that some expectancy of reward was not met. Schultz and colleagues have found that dopamine neurons show phasic activations when rewards occur unexpectedly or better than predicted, whereas they show phasic depressions when rewards are omitted or occur worse than predicted.[8] Importantly, dopamine neurons do not respond to fully predicted rewards. This suggests that dopamine represents a means of indicating an error in prediction, such that it demonstrates a discrepancy (or error) between what could be learned and what is currently learned.

Moreover, the dopamine response may serve even broader functions as well. It is likely that the dopamine response serves as a teaching signal concerning relevant stimuli in the environment. The concentration of dopamine neurons is relatively small but their projections reach a broad range of forebrain structures. These projections are believed to focus and enhance neurotransmitter signaling in the more-advanced forebrain. In this way, the release of dopamine in the forebrain would serve to direct attention towards stimuli in the environment that are currently associated with the foods we like. It is also likely that subsequent *plasticity* (physical changes in neurons) could serve to enhance this learning signal concerning associations between predictive stimuli and food. In short, this midbrain system is constantly *learning* about stimuli that predict food rewards and *teaching* the forebrain to pay more attention to them when they appear.

What this research means is that dopamine responds only to food rewards that are not fully predicted by some environmental cue. As an environmental cue comes to predict the occurrence of food rewards, dopamine neurons begin to increase their response rate to the predictive stimulus and actually decrease response rate when the reward is delivered. For example, say that you usually eat dinner at a certain time or with certain company. If this has become routine, then it is likely that dopamine will begin to respond at the time dinner usually occurs or when company arrives and will decrease when the dinner is actually served. This dopamine system is designed to anticipate the foods we like. If cues come to predict the occurrence of sweet-tasting, fatty foods, then the dopamine response will begin to send the "wanting" signal at the time the reward is predicted, not when it actually occurs. How many poor kids have had their hands swatted away from a piping hot dinner because it needed to cool? They smelled it, they saw it, and therefore they wanted it—darn that insatiable dopamine! You simply don't have to eat a food to want it when it is predicted by environmental cues such as smell and sight. This leaves the dieter in a dilemma because simply changing his or her diet will not stop the dopamine system from wanting the foods a person likes. There are only so many times we can resist a piping hot delicacy before we just give in and eat!

The Pleasurable Diet

The pleasurable diet is, of course, the one we would consume if it wouldn't make us so fat. My pleasurable diet is cold pizza or pastry for breakfast, an all-American cheeseburger and French fries for lunch, and some high-fat, high-carbohydrate pasta dish for dinner. It is the see-food diet, with no limitations. It is whatever diet we have learned to like and have tried to quit. The foods we eat on this diet cause very pleasurable increases in midbrain dopamine. Even if we stopped eating these foods, the dopamine response wouldn't stop.

When you are dieting, you still want and still like all the foods you have usually eaten. If you don't learn to like healthier foods, your diet will inevitably fail—this dopamine system will make sure of it. The reality is that we eat mostly for the pleasure or reward of it, not to eliminate some homeostatic hunger. Dopamine mediates the pleasure we take from eating and helps to ensure that any efforts to deviate from a pleasurable diet will be short-lived. At the start of a diet, you won't likely consume high-fat, sweet-tasting foods. But the dopamine system is sophisticated in its response to this. You don't have to consume such foods for dopamine to rise; all you need is to come into contact with cues that predict their consumption. Thus, you must make efforts to avoid seeing the foods, either on television or while grocery shopping. You must make efforts to discontinue any typical eating patterns such as when you eat (time), with whom you eat (people), or even where you eat (place), since all these stimuli can act as cues for dopamine release in the midbrain. Therefore, this dopamine response is involved as much in keeping you on your pleasurable diet as it is in helping you to take pleasure for being on the diet. This is a major reason why almost all cold-turkey diets fail, along with most diets in general. You simply cannot take for granted the physiological components of food reward responsible for making the foods you eat so pleasurable.

Still, this is the first of three reasons why shifting diets is so difficult—you may have noticed that there are three chapters in this section. Besides the fact that we *want* the foods that we *like*, we also have innate (or unlearned) likes for many foods that happen to be unhealthy, and innate dislikes for many foods that happen to be healthy. While this is indubitably linked to our dopamine response, it also has unique implications that will be discussed in the next chapter.

Notes

1. Hull, E. M. (2002). The nigrostriatal and mesolimbic dopamine tracts. In M. M. Slaughter (Ed.), *Basic Concepts in Neuroscience: A Student's Survival Guide* (pp. 187-208). New York: McGraw Hill.
2. Yun, I. A., Wakabayashi, K. T., Fields, H. L., & Nicola, S. M. (2004). The ventral tegmental area is required for the behavioral and nucleus accumbens neuronal firing responses to incentive cues. *Journal of Neuroscience, 24*, 2923-2933.
3. Kelley, A. E., & Berridge, K. C. (2002). The neuroscience of natural rewards: Relevance to addictive drugs. *The Journal of Neuroscience*, 22 (9), 3306-3311.
4. Wyvell, C. L., & Berridge, K. C. (2000). Intra-nucleus accumbens amphetamine increases the conditioned incentive salience of sucrose reward: enhancement of reward "wanting" without enhanced "liking" or response reinforcement. *Journal of Neuroscience, 20*, 8122–8130.
5. Tremblay, L., & Schultz, W. (1999). Relative reward preference in primate orbitofrontal cortex. *Nature*, 398 (6729), 704-708.
6. Pecina, S., & Berridge, K. C. (2000) Opioid eating site in nucleus accumbens shell mediates food intake and hedonic "liking": map based on microinjection Fos plumes. *Brain Research, 863*, 71–86.
7. Schultz, W. (2002). Getting formal with dopamine and reward. *Neuron*, 36 (2), 241-63.
8. Tobler, P. N., Dickinson, A., & Schultz, W. (2003). Coding of predicted reward omission by dopamine neurons in a conditioned inhibition paradigm. *Journal of Neuroscience, 23*, 10402-10410.

Chapter 5: Innate Likes and Dislikes

The human fetus consumes 200-760 milliliters of amniotic fluid daily, and that amniotic fluid contains many substances found in the very foods you enjoy today, including glucose, fructose, lactic acid, fatty acids, phospholipids, urea, amino acids, proteins, and salts, to name a few.[1] The human fetus is remarkably alert to and capable of learning about odors and tastes preterm. The taste buds are well developed (although not fully developed) at the beginning of the second trimester of pregnancy,[2] and the olfactory (smell) capabilities are functional early in the third trimester.[3] Thus, the equipment necessary to experience sensations of taste and smell is available preterm. Knowing this, researchers have sought to test hypotheses concerning the perceptual capabilities of human fetuses, and how their sensory experiences in utero affect their eating behavior. In this chapter we will review much of these researchers work and the implications their findings have for human diet.

Theories of Flavor Perception

A common belief among scientists is that humans have a genetic predisposition toward liking or disliking the tastes and flavors of the foods they consume. Yet to understand these predispositions, we must first define human flavor perception. Indeed, it has only been within the past decade or so that two mainstream theoretical models were developed to explain how we perceive taste. One describes that humans can only transduce four (possibly) five tastes, whereas a competing, but less-accepted theory suggests that the number of taste categories we perceive is potentially infinite.

The *across fiber pattern*, or *population theory*,[4,5] postulates a substantial number of taste categories (possibly more than we care to count, but more than four or five). It also purports that our perception of taste results from a synthesis of neural receptor activity such that it would be almost impossible to calculate the number of taste and odor combinations a person can perceive. This is used to explain why humans are not very good at describing the taste of food. For example, we commonly describe foods indirectly by saying they taste like this or that. It is rather difficult for us to specifically describe or identify the culinary subtleties of the foods we consume. Unfortunately, this model has received varying support, and therefore most research conducted on human taste perception follows the framework of another theory, which asserts instead that we can count the number of tastes we perceive on the fingers of one hand. Talk about two theories that couldn't be more different!

This theory, the *basic tastes theory*, emphasizes the limiting capacity for mammals, including humans, to experience and perceive tastes.[6,7] This theory purports that the four basic tastes—sweet, salty, sour, and bitter—are the only taste categories that exist, although this model does not discount the possibility that umami may also be a valid taste category. Umami, a taste arising from glutamate, is not always included as a basic taste, and further research will be needed to identify its neural receptor. The logic for this theory is fairly straightforward: Where are your *taste receptors* (also referred to as *taste buds*)? As you may already be aware, taste receptors are located on the tongue. Therefore, for a substance to be a taste, it must be able to activate one of the taste receptors on the tongue. If a receptor for any given taste is not identified on the tongue, then it can't be a taste. To date, only four unique taste receptors have been definitively identified: salty, sour, bitter, and sweet. Again, umami is likely to be added as a fifth taste, but for now little is known about its receptor and its *innate* (unlearned) qualities. Therefore, for the purposes of this discussion, we perceive only four tastes; anything else is an odor.

Our perception of taste regulates eating by providing information to discrete brain regions concerning how good or bad a food tastes. Humans innately prefer salty and sweet-tasting foods; humans innately dislike sour and bitter tastes. All naturally occurring poisons are bitter, and sour fruits are not ripe and provide less nutrition. How humans perceive the taste of food is surprisingly not well known. Molecules within food dissolve in saliva and activate one of four receptor types on the tongue. Each receptor type provides information about a food—sweetness indicates safety in nature, such as the ripeness of fruits; salt provides needed sodium; bitter indicates poisonous foods; and sour indicates spoiled foods. Also, the types of chemicals that activate these receptors are known, but the pathways (to the brain) for these receptors have been difficult to identify. Receptors that detect salt are most effectively activated by sodium chloride (NaCl). Those that detect sour are most effectively activated by hydrogen ions present in acid solutions. Those that detect bitter are most effectively activated by an alkaloid such as quinine; and a sugar molecule (as you may have guessed) most effectively activates receptors that detect sweetness.

Gustatory processing (processing of the molecules we can taste) is so important that information about taste is transmitted via three of our twelve cranial nerves—that's a quarter of the cranial nerves partly responsible for keeping the brain informed of what is going on in the body. In case you are interested, the cranial nerves of which I am speaking are numbers 7 (anterior tongue), 9 (posterior tongue), and 10 (palate and epiglottis). Taste information is relayed via the nucleus of the solitary tract (medulla) and into the brain regions responsible for perceiving taste—the primary gustatory cortex (identifying the taste cue), amygdala (for emotional components of the taste cue), and the hypothalamus (activates peripheral responses that cause behavioral, metabolic, hormonal, and neural changes to enable us to seek and consume food).

The basic tastes theory makes four important statements. First, any oral perception that is not a basic taste is not a taste at all (nongustatory). This means that unless it is salty, sour, bitter, or sweet, you smell it and do not taste it. This includes flavors many people refer to as *tastes* such as banana, almond, strawberry, maple, and so on. Second, basic tastes are distinct and can be recognized when mixed with other tastes, with few exceptions. As it turns out, humans are pretty good at identifying the tastes of different foods. Third, the physiological mechanisms underlying our perception of tastes are also distinct, such that each taste has its own designated receptor, and this receptor *transduces*—converts a physical stimulus such as a sugar molecule into an electrical impulse—information via specific neural pathways. Again, while the specific pathways have not been clearly identified, it is most likely that the taste receptors on our tongues do follow identifiable neural pathways. Fourth, the intensity of tastes relative to other tastes determines its perceptual salience, such that weaker tastes are considered less meaningful and described as *side tastes*.[8]

Thus, this model establishes that only four (possibly five) tastes truly exist and that any other "taste" is perceived only with the bolstering of other sensory systems, especially olfaction (smell). Tastes can be distinguished from other tastes, with exceptions, and the concentration level of tastes determines our ability to perceive them. What this means is that every flavor we perceive comes to be liked or disliked via its association with the only cues we truly taste—salty, sour, bitter, sweet, and possibly umami. If we drink a sweet-tasting banana drink, then we tend to consume more banana-flavored drinks; if we eat a bitter-tasting apple and become sick, we may never consume an apple-flavored food or drink again. Thus, most flavors associated with the diets we prefer have been learned and there is no evidence we ever stop learning.

As implied in this model, our chemical senses—specifically sense of smell—have somewhat permissive effects on flavor perception. The sense of smell is initiated when odorants bind with olfactory receptors located on cilia in the nasal cavity. There are two routes by which we can smell: orthonasal and retronasal. The latter route is understood to play a significant role in flavor perception,[9] and its diminished effectiveness over time is partly responsible for the loss of flavor perception as we age.[10] *Orthonasal perception* is via the nostrils; *retronasal perception* occurs when odors travel toward the roof of the nasal cavity in the back of the throat. Retronasal odor perception occurs whenever we eat, and contributes to how we "taste" the subtleties of the foods we consume.

If your retronasal perception were blocked (e.g., by a stuffed-up nose), you would probably be unable to sense subtle qualities of the foods you eat. Thus, without the ability to smell, we are left with only the bland taste qualities of that food. All the subtle odors that add to the flavor of the food would be lost. Most people report experiencing this and the experience is consistent with the basic tastes model which attributes any "tastes" we sense other than the basic tastes to the combination of taste and odor. This has important implications for what we learn about food, since likes or dislikes for certain tastes are innate; they do not require learning. Therefore, it is very likely that every odor or flavor you like or dislike—other than salty, sour, bitter, and sweet—was learned because of its association with taste cues. This means that the majority of the likes and dislikes that make up your diet can be modified through learning and experience. The following section shows how researchers came to understand which tastes are liked and disliked without learning.

Innate Likes and Dislikes

Tastes appear to be prenatally liked (e.g., sweet) or disliked (e.g., sour) by the human fetus, although taste buds are not fully mature until about forty days following birth. Specific stereotypical facial responses from newborns are used to measure such likes and dislikes. Infants tend to respond positively to sweet tastes with sucking movements and facial relaxation, whereas they react negatively to bitter and sour tastes with facial protrusions and grimaces.[11] Salt, on the other hand, elicits no stereotypical facial response from a fetus—and therefore no preference—although infants within two hours after birth can distinguish between saltiness and the other basic tastes. Findings such as these strongly suggest that taste stimuli are innately liked or disliked preterm, although it will become exceedingly evident that later learning can modify the innate qualities of these basic tastes (i.e., salty, sour, bitter, sweet).

Salt. Perhaps the most physiologically important taste is that of saltiness. Sodium is arguably the most sought-after *cation* (positively charged ion) in the human body. Sufficient sodium levels are necessary to maintain appropriate distribution of water and osmotic pressure surrounding our cells.[12] Concentrations of salt are constantly being balanced in the fluid compartments surrounding the cells in our bodies. If salt concentrations are too high, our cells die of thirst; if they become too low, our cells essentially die from drowning. Newborns are typically indifferent to the taste of salt within the first few months of birth, although this depends partly on fetal learning.[13] The earliest reliable preferences for salt have been suggested at about four months of age, presumably due to maturation of an infant's sensitivity to sodium.[14] These preferences are considered innate since four-month-old infants prefer the taste of salt even without prior experience with the taste. Thus, this shift at four months is believed to result from sensory maturation, not learning. Following this period, these innate preferences are modified primarily through learned dietary experiences. For example, infants who are kept on low-sodium diets (e.g., breast feeding) beyond six months of age tend to prefer low-sodium foods, whereas infants fed salty foods beyond six months of age acquire a stronger preference for the taste of salt.[15] Still, amniotic experiences can enhance preferences for salt by the fetus.

A few studies report that children of mothers who experienced moderate vomiting during pregnancy express taste aversions (dislikes) to salt, whereas infants from mothers who experienced severe vomiting show taste preferences for salt following birth.[16] (The reason for this is explained in the chapter 6 introduction.) This suggests that innate preferences for salt can be modified even before birth. In other words, the preference or aversion to salt expressed by an infant seems to be dependent on the child's amniotic experiences as a fetus, possibly since the environment of the amnion is perceived by the infant to predict the external environment. In fact, some research suggests that these amniotic experiences influence long-term, lifelong salt intake in humans.[17]

Sweet. On the other hand, sweet-tasting solutions, such as sucrose and saccharin, are preferred prenatally. When term and preterm (33-40 weeks postconception) infants are given a choice between a latex nipple and a sweetened nipple (e.g., a sucrose-flavored gelatin nipple), both groups of infants suck more often and more intensely on the sweetened nipple.[18] This sucking response is commonly used as a measurement for preferences in infants, such that greater sucking of a sweetened nipple would suggest a preference for the sweetened taste on that nipple. Since both term and preterm infants respond preferentially to sweet tastes, these preferences must be occurring prenatally. Also, these preferences are marked before postnatal learning can occur; thus sweet tastes are considered innately preferred by humans, although these preferences do appear to diminish with age, probably resulting from maturational shifts during adolescence.

Bitter. In general, humans do not prefer bitter tastes (e.g., urea and quinine), although they are typically indifferent to the taste within hours of delivery.[19] Despite their indifference to bitterness immediately following labor, they do consistently reject bitter-tasting solutions within a few days postnatal.[20] The transductory pathways involved in the detection of bitter tastes is very complicated, since a variety of compounds can activate taste receptors for bitterness. Possibly the intricate mechanisms involved in the detection of bitterness are not fully responsive to its presence until a few days postnatal. This would suggest that these transductory pathways require postnatal maturation, and could explain why infants fail to respond to bitterness until days following birth.

Sour. Alternatively, infants do noticeably reject sour tastes such as citric acid at birth, with no delay in responsiveness, suggesting that this taste is innately disliked. Further observations have found that infants continue to respond negatively to sour tastes at four months postnatal, as measured by facial expressions,[21] and no evidence appears to contradict these findings.

The Calming Taste of Sweet: Implications for Addiction

What this evidence means is that the basic tastes are liked or disliked without learning. This also means that there must be a brain system (or systems) innately designed to respond to these tastes, and this has particularly important implications for the tastes we like (specifically sweetness)—enter the dopamine system. As it turns out, a sweet-tasting solution can do more than just taste sweet. Infants actually can be calmed and find relief from pain following ingestion of a sweet-tasting solution. For example, when a sweet-tasting liquid (e.g., water mixed with glucose or table sugar) is administered on the tongue of an infant prior to a heel prick (which causes pain), this significantly reduces infant crying time.[22] Many hospitals now use this strategy to reduce discomfort and pain when taking blood samples from newborn infants. Placing drops of water in the mouth of an infant has no effect; only when the water is sweetened is the calming effect observed. Even a mother's breast milk (which tastes moderately sweet), consumed during breast-feeding prior to a heel prick, is not as effective as a strong sweet-tasting sucrose solution.[23] Various concentrations of sweet-tasting sucrose, fructose, and glucose can effectively elicit this *analgesic* (pain relieving) effect in infants[24] and research suggests that these effects are apparently specific to the sweet-tasting properties of these sugars.[25] Since consuming these sugars significantly calms both term and preterm infants, it is most likely that the sweetness-mediated calming effect is functional before birth.[26]

To better understand how sweet solutions could produce these effects, researchers have looked at the neurochemical pathways involved in taste perception. What they have found is that the taste of sweetness on the tongue triggers a nerve impulse that goes to the brain and activates the same system responsible for drug addiction. Specifically, sweet tastes activate opioid chemicals in the midbrain, which produces the calming effects in infants. This opioid release in turn triggers the release of dopamine in this same brain region, which makes the taste of sweet feel very rewarding—this is the same dopamine system discussed in chapter 4. These chemicals (opioids and dopamine) are released in response to the intake of many classes of drugs including heroin and morphine, which are very addictive. This has sparked a great deal of controversy, since it leads to a very interesting question: can the neurobiological effects of sweet-taste ingestion and drug use interact?

Consider that constant exposure to these endogenous opioids—those produced by our bodies—eliminates the effectiveness of sweet tastes in producing analgesia.[27] This may explain why sweetness is ineffective at calming an infant conceived by a heroin-addicted mother. Presumably the opioid system was overstimulated during pregnancy by the heroin the mother was using. Thus, the relatively lesser level of opioid increase caused by the sweetness no longer had an effect. What this also means is that increased drug use by a mother can decrease an infant's responsiveness to sweetness at birth. This may lead to increased preference for sweetness later in life—since more sweetness must be consumed to produce the rewarding dopamine effect. Also, increased consumption of sweetened water in the first few months of life can result in greater preference for the taste of sweetness by two years of age.[28] If increased intake of sweetness and heroin causes a very similar opioid-dopamine response in the midbrain, then both may have the same long-term effects: both may in later life increase preference for and therefore consumption of foods that taste sweet.

It is also the case that anything associated with this calming response is subject to learning—infants will express preference for persons who give them the calming sweet taste.[29] In fact, over time, they are dependent on these associations in order for the sweet taste to be effectively calming—the ability of sweet-tasting solutions to calm infants fades periodically during early postnatal development. Immediately following labor, infants are successfully calmed by various concentrations of sweet-tasting solutions. Yet, at about four weeks, sucrose is effective at alleviating crying only when administered (or paired) with some other form of sensory stimulation, such as eye contact by the administrator,[30] sucking on a pacifier,[31] or the physical touch of being held.[32] At about nine weeks of age, infants are calmed by sucrose, but this effect lasts only seconds. At about twelve weeks, neither eye contact nor sucrose is effective,[33] although allowing infants to suck on a pacifier remains effective for a while longer.[34] Thus, in time, this effect eventually dulls, likely due to the brain's ability over time to learn to tolerate the increased opioid and dopamine release.

An equally intriguing question is about how this influences our tendencies toward drug addiction. If early drug use can increase a person's intake of sweetened foods and drinks later in life, then it could be the case that early intake of sweets will increase drug intake or tendencies toward drug addiction later in life. While to date, this suggestion has little direct scientific evidence to support or reject such a possibility, it is not beyond scientific reason to suggest that there is a link between the tastes and drugs that stimulate the *same* brain regions and neurotransmitters. It is known that the ventral dopamine system does not discriminate among sensory inputs; whether we eat it, swallow it, or inject it, the dopamine response will behave as if it likes and wants it. After all, this system "behaves" as though anything capable of stimulating it must be needed for life, regardless of whether this is true. This is (in part) why many scientists today believe that our diets can be *addictive* even though (unlike addictive drugs) food is *needed* to sustain life.

Training Our Taste Buds

Despite the implications for the probable addictive qualities of the basic tastes, almost every facet of our diets is learned and can therefore be modified. Although it is clear that the basic tastes are innately preferred or rejected even before birth, our preference or rejection of all other odors and flavors is the result of experience; i.e., we learn about them. Anything we like that does not stimulate our taste buds, we must learn about—including flavors commonly described as tastes, such as strawberry, banana, almond, cherry, and so on. Odors mixed with sweet-tasting foods come to be liked; odors mixed with bitter-tasting foods can come to be disliked. For example, the smell of coffee in the morning is rejuvenating for those who have learned to like it—likely due to adding sugars and high-fat creamers. Even our innate likes and dislikes for the basic tastes are subject to learning. For example, we learn to like the bitter taste of coffee by mixing it with sweeteners. Chocolate is very bitter and probably wouldn't be consumed if it weren't for the sugar added to make it taste sweet. In all, this means that you can modify your diet and learn to like it, even prefer it.

This is great news for people tired of short-lived dieting solutions for a long-term body. However, this statement comes with a caveat: likes (and some dislikes) for non-tastes take time to be acquired—although learning can be effective in as little as three to ten sittings. The key is that we must essentially "train" our taste buds—and the brain regions that these taste buds stimulate—to like new and healthier foods and flavors. In the next chapter we will discuss one last factor making it difficult to shift our liking to less preferred foods: *mere exposure*. Basically, the more often we consume a food, the more we eat of it, and the more we like it. Of course, we have the greatest exposure to the foods in our traditional diet—you know, the diet that many of us are trying to change.

Notes

1. Liley, A. W. (1972). Disorders of amniotic fluid. In N. S. Assali (Ed.), *Pathophysiology of gestation: fetal placental disorders, Vol. 2* (pp. 157-206). San Diego, CA: Academic Press.
2. Bradley, R. M. (1972). Development of the taste bud and gustatory papillae in human fetuses. In J. F. Bosma (Ed.), *The third symposium on oral sensation and perception: The mouth of the infant* (pp. 137-162). Springfield, Ill: Charles C. Thomas.
3. Pihet, S., Mellier, D., Bullinger, A., & Schaal, B. (1997). Reponses comportementales aux odeurs chez le nouveau-ne premature: Etude preliminaire [Behavioral responses of preterm newborns to odors: Preliminary study]. *Enfance, 1*, 33-46.
4. Halpern, B. P. (1997). Psychophysics of taste. In G. K. Beauchamp & L. M. Bartoshuk (Eds.), *Taste and Smelling: Handbook of Perception and Cognition* (2nd ed., pp. 77-123). San Diego: Academic Press.
5. Halpern, B. P. (1999). Taste. In R. A. Wilson & F. Keil (Eds.), *The MIT Encyclopedia of the Cognitive Sciences* (pp. 826-828). Cambridge: Bradford Books.
6. Halpern, B. P. (2002). Taste. In H. Pashler & S. Yantis (Eds.), *Stevens' Handbook of Experimental Psychology, Vol. 1* (3rd ed., pp. 653-690). New York: John Wiley & Sons, Inc.
7. Lawless, H. T. (2000). Taste. In E. B. Goldstein (Ed.), *Blackwell Handbook of Perception* (pp. 601-635). Malden, MA: Blackwell.
8. Frank, M. E. (2000). Neuron types, receptors, behavior, and taste quality. *Physiology and Behavior, 69*, 53-62.
9. Rozin, P. (1982). "Taste-smell confusions" and the duality of the olfactory sense. *Perception and Psychophysics, 31*, 397-401.
10. Tuorila, H., Niskanen, T., & Maunuksela, E. (2001). Perception and pleasantness of a food with varying odor and flavor among the elderly and young. *Journal of Nutrition, Health & Aging, 5* (4), 266-268.
11. Rosenstein, D., & Oster, H. (1988). Differential facial responses to four basic tastes in newborns. *Child Development, 59* (6), 1555-1568.
12. McCaughey, S. A., & Scott, T. R. (1998). The taste of sodium. *Neuroscience and Biobehavioral Reviews, 22*, 663-676.

13. Crook, C. K. (1978). Taste perception in the newborn infant. *Infant Behavior and Development, 1*, 52-69.
14. Harris, G., Thomas, A., & Booth, D. A. (1990). Development of salt taste in infancy. *Developmental Psychology, 26* (4), 534-538.
15. Mennella, J. A., & Beauchamp, G. K. (1996). The early development of human flavor preferences. In E. D. Capaldi (Ed.), *Why We Eat What We Eat: The Psychology of Eating.* Washington, DC: American Psychological Association.
16. Beauchamp, G. K., Cowart, B. J., Mennella, J. A., & Marsh, R. R. (1994). Infant salt taste: Developmental, methodological, and contextual factors. *Developmental Psychobiology, 27* (6), 353-365.
17. Leshem, M. (1998). Salt preference in adolescence is predicted by common prenatal and infantile mineralofluid loss. *Physiology & Behavior, 63* (4), 699-704.
18. Maone, T. R., Mattes, R. D., Bernbaum, J. C., & Beauchamp, G. K. (1990). A new method for delivering a taste without fluids to preterm and term infants. *Developmental Psychobiology, 23*, 179-191.
19. Desor, J. A., Maller, O., & Andrews, K. (1975). Ingestive responses of human newborns to salty, sour and bitter stimuli. *Journal of Comparative and Physiological Psychology, 89*, 966-970.
20. Kajiura, H., Cowart, B. J., & Beauchamp, G. K. (1992). Early developmental changes in bitter taste responses in human infants. *Developmental Psychobiology, 25*, 375-386.
21. Bennett, D. S., Bendersky, M., & Lewis, M. (2002). Facial expressivity at 4 months: A context by expression analysis. *Infancy, 3* (1), 97-113.
22. Eriksson, M., Gradin, M., & Schollin, J. (1999). Oral glucose and venepuncture reduce blood sampling pain in newborns. *Early Human Development, 55* (3), 211-218.
23. Bilgen, H., Oezek, E., Cebeci, D., & Oers, R. (2001). Comparison of sucrose, expressed breast milk, and breast-feeding on the neonatal response to heel prick. *Journal of Pain, 2* (5), 301-305.
24. Blass, E. M., & Smith, B. A. (1992). Differential effects of sucrose, fructose, glucose, and lactose on crying in 1- to 3-day-old human infants: Qualitative and quantitative considerations. *Developmental Psychology, 28* (5), 804-810.
25. Barr, R. G., Pantel, M. S., Young, S. N., Wright, J. H., Hendricks, L. A., & Gravel, R. (1999). The response of crying newborns to sucrose: Is it a "sweetness" effect? *Physiology & Behavior, 66* (3), 409-417.
26. Smith, B. A., & Blass, E. M. (1996). Taste-mediated calming in premature, preterm, and full-term human infants. *Developmental Psychology, 32* (6), 1084-1089.
27. Smith, B. A., Stevens, K., Torgerson, W. S., & Kim, J. H. (1992). Diminished reactivity of postmature human infants to sucrose compared with term infants. *Developmental Psychology, 28* (5), 811-820.
28. Beauchamp, G.K., & Moran, M. (1985). Acceptance of sweet and salty taste in 2-year-old children. *Appetite, 5*, 291-305.
29. Blass, E. M., & Camp, C. A. (2001). The ontogeny of face recognition: Eye contact and sweet taste induce face preference in 9- and 12-week-old human infants. *Developmental Psychology, 37* (6), 762-774.
30. Zeifman, D., Delaney, S., & Blass, E. M. (1996). Sweet taste, looking, and calm in 2- and 4-week-old infants: The eyes have it. *Developmental Psychology, 32* (6), 1090-1099.

31. Akman, I., Ozek, E., Bilgen, H., Ozdogan, T., & Cebeci, D. (2002). Sweet solutions and pacifiers for pain relief in newborn infants. *Journal of Pain*, 3 (3), 199-202.
32. Gormally, S., Barr, R. G., Wertheim, L., Alkawaf, R., Calinoiu, N., & Young, S. N. (2001). Contact and nutrient caregiving effects on newborn infant pain responses. *Developmental Medicine & Child Neurology*, 43 (1), 28-38.
33. Blass, E. M. (1998). Changing influence of sucrose and visual engagement in 2- 12-week-old infants: Implications for maternal face recognition. *Infant Behavior and Development*, 20, 423-434.
34. Blass, E. M., & Camp, C. A. (2003). Changing determinants of crying termination in 6- to 12-week-old human infants. *Developmental Psychobiology*, 42 (3), 312-316.

Chapter 6: Mere Exposure Learning

The human fetus is exposed to a variety of taste and odor molecules originating from the mother, most of them in the amniotic fluid. The odor of the amniotic fluid is of great importance to human feeding since it reflects the foods that the expectant mother has eaten.[1] Not surprisingly, researchers have used amniotic samples to gather evidence concerning fetal learning in the *amnion* (fetal environment). Findings reported in major psychological journals demonstrate many characteristics of fetal learning. One explanation for neonatal learning is referred to as *mere exposure*. Mere exposure is a form of learning in which no apparent reinforcer is used to increase the probability of a behavior, and this learning continues through the human lifespan. Through mere exposure, a fetus learns to recognize and prefer the flavors associated with the mother's diet. This form of learning is mediated by simple exposure—familiarity appears to be enough to facilitate flavor preferences even before birth.

Mere exposure has important implications for learning. First, it is important that we can learn what foods and flavors are safe to eat. One mechanism for our brain to judge this is to monitor those foods we consume repeatedly without ill consequence. The more I eat a food without getting sick, the more confident I become that the food is safe to eat. Again, in the course of evolution, we did not have the Food and Drug Administration (FDA) to assist us in making these judgments. Instead, we had to learn through experience. Our ability to learn through mere exposure is a testament to the body's effort to increase liking for foods that are safe to eat—and therefore the probability of consuming these foods.

Second, it would make sense for learning by mere exposure to begin preterm. Consider that a fetus spends up to 40 weeks in an environment rich with the odors and tastes consumed by the mother. If fetuses can perceive these tastes and odors (which they can), then it would be useful for them to acquire preferences for these flavors as well. This is because the mother is consuming these tastes and odors without ill consequence. The fetus can essentially infer what flavors are safe to consume in the world by monitoring the flavors that their mother consumes.

For example (as first mentioned in chapter 5), some women experience frequent vomiting during pregnancy. Vomiting results in significant loss of minerals and fluids, including deprivational levels of salt, for mother and fetus. This deprivation of salt in the amnion influences the fetus's preferences for salt following birth. Researchers have compared 16-week-old infants of mothers who reported little or no vomiting during pregnancy, with infants of mothers who reported frequent or severe vomiting.[2] The results indicate that infants whose mothers experienced little or no vomiting during pregnancy consumed lesser amounts of salty solutions (aversive response), relative to infants from mothers experiencing frequent vomiting bouts during pregnancy (preferential response). These results not only suggest that preferences or aversions to tastes can be acquired or even modified in utero; they also suggest that the amnion represents to the baby what the world is like.

The human body is bathed in saltwater at a concentration that must be balanced for the cells to live. Therefore, acquiring sodium from the environment is very important to survival. For the fetus, if the mother vomits frequently, there will be little salt in the amnion. This would indicate to the child that the environment into which he or she will be born is also sodium-deprived. Therefore, it would be good for the baby to increase preference for salt in what he or she expects to be a low-sodium world, so that the child makes sure to consume it when he or she comes across it. This may be why infants express greater preference for salt if they were deprived of this taste in utero. Regardless, this indicates that a fetus can learn about the tastes their mother consumes.

Flavor Learning at Birth

A fetus can learn about diet. As indicated in the introduction, there is convincing evidence that we begin acquiring our dietary preferences preterm. For example, researchers have investigated preterm preferences by having some expectant mothers consume anise-flavored substances late into pregnancy, while another group of expectant mothers did not.[3] When the mother consumed the odorous substance, the fetus presumably could smell the anise in the amniotic fluid. Thus, the researchers hypothesized that the fetus could learn to prefer this odor prenatally simply by exposure to it during fetal development. To test this, a sample of newborns at a median age of only 8 postnatal hours, and again at 4 days, were placed face up with two odors suspended above them, one to the left and the other to the right of each newborn. The researchers hypothesized that the newborns would *prefer*—orient their heads to whichever side an odor was located—the flavor to which they had been exposed prenatally. This test showed that newborns exposed prenatally to the anise odor did orient their heads toward it for a longer duration than they did toward a neutral odor—thus, they expressed a preference for the anise odor. Newborns not exposed to the anise flavor prenatally showed no preference for either odor. Thus, the fetus can experience and learn about the odors of foods that a mother eats; results similar to this have been readily replicated. For example, studies also have shown that infants will prefer garlic-flavored solutions that were consumed by their mothers during pregnancy.[4,5] These reports strongly suggest that the unique olfactory environment experienced by a fetus has a seemingly profound impact on the later establishment of dietary odor preferences.

Labor enhances learning. Experiments conducted by Varendi and colleagues in 2002 demonstrated how these preferences are acquired.[6] They tested thirty-one newborns, all of whom were delivered by cesarean section. Fifteen of these subjects were delivered following uterine contractions, i.e., labor experienced by their mothers. The infants of the mothers who had experienced labor were compared with the infants from the mothers who had not experienced labor. Within one hour after birth, the researchers exposed each newborn to one of two odors—cherry or passion fruit—referred to as the exposure odor. The newborns were tested at a median age of 80 hours. The researchers placed the subjects face up and suspended the two odors, one to the left and the other to the right of each newborn. Half the newborns in each group had been exposed to the cherry, the other half to passion fruit. The researchers expected the newborns to *prefer* the flavor to which they had previous exposure. The findings showed that infants born following labor showed significant preference (or a positive head orientation) for the exposure odor, whereas the non-labor infants failed to show significant preference for either odor. This indicates that an infant's ability to learn about odors in the environment is enhanced by contractions. Thus, contractions—which prior to modern medicine were required for successful labor—acted as a trigger for learning. This trigger appears to heighten the infant's awareness of the environment at the most appropriate time—as the child enters the world. In addition, it appears that the longer a mother experiences contractions, the longer the infant will orient to the odor he or she experiences within an hour of birth. With greater exposure, newborns express greater preference for the odors they experience during their first hour postnatal.

How might the brain be able to accomplish this? Evidence suggests that contractions apparently increase norepinephrine release in the fetus, thereby enhancing the fetus's alertness to its environment and the odors in it. Norepinephrine is a neurotransmitter that is synthesized and released in the brain—specifically in the locus coeruleus—and plays a primary role in facilitating attention. Thus, its release at the time of labor appears to be associated with an enhanced ability for a fetus to learn about the odors in the environment by enhancing how aware the infant is of its environment, including an awareness of the mother's odorous signature—and even the mother's voice.[7]

Learning involves the acquisition of preferences, not neophobia. Neophobia is defined as a reluctance to consume a novel or unfamiliar solution. The experiments presented thus far draw attention to the salient sensory capabilities of a fetus in the amnion. These findings are consistent with the notion that a fetus can recognize and learn to prefer odors that originate from its mother. Whether researchers tested an infant's preference for an odor experienced in utero, or immediately following birth, the results were the same: preferences were established. Yet, how do we know the infants prefer these odors per se? Is it possible they simply avoid non-familiar odors (a neophobic response)?

To answer this question, researchers have used a mother's amniotic fluid to test preferences.[8] In one study, infants were separated into two conditions contingent on whether they were breast-fed or bottle-fed. Three-day-old infants, both breast-fed and bottle-fed, showed preferences for familiar amniotic fluid (fAF) in this study. They oriented their heads for a longer duration toward the amniotic fluid of their mothers—relative to non-familiar amniotic fluid (nfAF). In later experiments, they compared fAF and nfAF with a control solution (gauze dampened with 20 drops of distilled water). Infants in all groups still showed preference for the odor of fAF relative to both controls, suggesting that the preferences established in the initial experiments were the result of a positive orientation toward the fAF, and not an avoidance of the nfAF. In other words, infants learned to prefer its smell, not avoid other, non-familiar odors.

Additional research has revealed that this preference is so robust that bottle-fed infants even prefer the odor of AF to the odor of their formula milk.[9] Studies on breast milk odors have revealed that the odor of flavors (such as garlic and vanilla) consumed by mothers can be detected in their breast milk, and that these flavors are later preferred by a newborn.[10] Additionally, mothers who change their diet soon after pregnancy—and thus change the olfactory cues familiar to the baby—report an increased difficulty in establishing breast-feeding.[11] Studies such as these clearly indicate that a fetus not only learns about the odors the mother consumes, but specifically learns to prefer these odors.

Breast or Bottle?

Many mothers have experienced the cognitive dissonance regarding the decision to breast-feed or bottle-feed their infants. Certainly, as an infant matures, the child's sensory world is enhanced. This makes an infant's eating experiences more convoluted, yet bolsters the baby's opportunity to learn about the flavors and foods in his or her diet. Infants can express preferences by way of facial responses to sweet-tasting solutions as young as nine weeks old.[12] As they grow into mid to late childhood, babies' abilities to differentiate and analyze a combination of taste mixtures become evident.[13] As an infant develops through childhood and into adulthood, the experiences that come with aging significantly influence the eating habits and patterns that are established. An infant's first feeding experience outside the mother's womb is, of course, via its mother's breast or a bottle. Yet, what is the impact of a mother's decision to bottle-feed or breast-feed on the infant's learning environment? Do infants learn about tastes and odors differently depending on how their mothers feed them? Can preferences resulting from early feeding be modified by later experience?

Mothers commonly make the decision to breast-feed or not based on a variety of factors including cost of formula, income level, cigarette use, regularity of doctor visits, age, and diet.[14,15] Since breast-feeding typically takes longer per session than bottle-feeding, breast-fed infants spend longer periods of time with their mothers. This mother-infant bonding may be one of the reasons breast-feeding mothers report less stress and more positive emotions than mothers who bottle-feed.[16] In terms of diet acquisition, one of the greatest advantages to breast-feeding is that the newborn can become more familiar with both the odors of the mother and the flavors in her breast milk associated with her diet. Recent reports indicate that the enhanced odorous environment of a breast-fed infant increases the infant's attentiveness to and interaction with the environment.[17] Whether an infant is breast-fed or bottle-fed, he or she undoubtedly can recognize and form preferences for the flavors consumed in early feeding.

Many compounds, such as tastes and odors, are transferred from a mother's diet to her milk. These compounds, most of which stimulate sense of smell, are often used to research early feeding in infants. In one study, two experiments—one with breast-fed infants and the other with bottle-fed infants—investigated how infants responded to a flavor change in milk or formula.[18] This study found that breast-fed infants exposed to vanilla flavors breast-fed longer and consumed more milk than those who were not exposed to the flavor. Although this change in behavior indicated a preference for vanilla, the researchers in this study point out that other factors, such as changes in the mothers' odors, could have influenced this observed change in behavior as well.

In a second experiment, similar results were observed in bottle-fed infants. Bottle-fed infants sucked more intently and spent more time feeding when the formula was vanilla-flavored relative to ordinary formula. These researchers suggest that the addition of a flavor, such as vanilla, to an otherwise bland diet may act to stimulate sucking behavior in infants, thereby facilitating breast- and bottle-feeding. Additionally, considering that flavors transfer from a mother's diet to her milk, they suggest that an advantage to breast-feeding may be that it gives the infant a first-hand experience with the flavors of foods consumed by his or her mother, family, and culture. It would be very difficult to accomplish this using formula milk. This suggestion is rather intuitive in light of the mounting evidence indicating that neonatal preferences for tastes and odors are observed years later in children and adults.[19] It is not a coincidence that most Italians seem to prefer Italian sausage and most Poles prefer Polish sausage—culture-specific foods are among those to which we have the greatest exposure, even before birth.

More proximate studies have tested whether early-infant preferences can be observed in children. These studies show that children who were bottle-fed as infants express flavor preferences in infancy and also in years following their last exposure to the formula. Formulas consumed by infants have been characterized in three classes: milk, soy (bitter-tasting), and hydrolysate (primarily sour-tasting) formulas.[20,21] Children fed protein hydrolysate formulas during infancy were more likely to prefer sour-tasting solutions than children who were fed milk formulas. Children fed soy formulas as infants showed stronger preferences for bitter-tasting solutions compared with controls. Thus, we are even more willing to consume tastes that we innately dislike (i.e., sour and bitter) simply because we were exposed to them during infancy. Preferences for sweet tastes were apparent in all children tested between four and seven years of age, but the strength of observed preferences was a function of the level of exposure children had with sugars, such that greater exposure to sugars resulted in stronger preferences for sweet-tasting solutions. Stated simply: merely being exposed to tastes we innately like in infancy can significantly affect *how much* we like and consume these tastes years later.

The *hedonic* (pleasure-seeking) behaviors of infants may be largely influenced by whether a child is breast-fed or bottle-fed. Clearly, breast milk provides a child not only with its mother's odorous signature, but also with the flavors of foods specific to its mother's diet and culture. Bottle-feeding on the other hand does have one major advantage: the infant has the opportunity to be fed by the father in many cases. Unfortunately, very little is known about a father's impact on an infant's early feeding experiences since most research on this topic has focused on mother-infant feeding. A mother usually wants to make an informed decision about the type of feeding best for her child. Of course, the mother provides a newborn with its first exposure to tastes and odors, and the resulting experiences will have lasting effects on later learning. Bottle-feeding typically limits the range of exposure of infants to different tastes and odors, while breast-feeding optimally exposes a child to the various tastes and odors consumed by its mother. In the end, though, either feeding alternative will give a child valuable experiences from which to learn about tastes and odors, and both will affect what the child chooses to eat later in life—for good and bad.

Flavor Learning in Adulthood

The mere exposure effect is not limited to infants. Mere exposure has been demonstrated to increase food preferences in children and adults as well. For example, researchers presented six children, all two-year-olds, with 20, 15, 10, 5, or 2 exposures to five initially novel cheeses, and presented eight two-year-olds with 20, 15, 10, 5, or 0 exposures to five initially novel fruits over a series of familiarization trials.[22] The children were given ten choice trials in which they could consume the experimental foods. The results clearly indicate that subjects increasingly consumed foods with which they were more familiar, producing an exposure frequency. Thus, the more mere exposure children had with the cheeses and fruits, the more they ate of them during the choice trials. Similar findings were observed in undergraduate students presented with 20, 10, 5, or 0 exposures to previously novel tropical fruit juices.[23] Again, a strong exposure effect was demonstrated, such that the more frequently a juice was tasted, the more it was liked (i.e., increased preference).

This research explains why certain aspects of our diets are difficult to eliminate. For example, consider how long your exposure has been to sweet-tasting and fatty foods. If you are like most people (and being honest), you probably have been consuming these foods since before birth. Of course, that's not entirely the individual's fault. All humans have an innate preference for the taste of sweet, and—as noted in chapter 4—fatty foods are very rewarding as well. Since mere exposure learning is evident into adulthood, our preferences for these foods increase as we continue to consume them. This means our preference for the sweet, fatty foods we consume every day continues to grow with each exposure. Even without innate preferences, mere exposure would seem too difficult to overcome. Most people have a significant history of mere exposure to foods they like and relatively less exposure to foods they dislike. Say, for example, you wanted to consume more bitter-tasting vegetables, such as broccoli and asparagus. Since bitter-tasting foods are innately disliked, it is unlikely you have had nearly the exposure to them as you have had to sweet-tasting, fatty foods. In órder for you to learn to prefer these bitter-tasting vegetables through mere exposure, you would have to catch up at least with the level of exposure you have had to other, more innately preferred foods. If learning were dependent on mere exposure alone, it would be difficult if not impossible to shift away from diets to which we have been exposed and which we have been consuming for life.

This is a good example of why people tend to cheat or quit diets altogether—we prefer flavors we have the greatest exposure to. It will always be the case that we have greater exposure to our pleasurable diet than to any new diet plan. We simply have greater exposure to the foods we have consumed since birth, and therefore greater preference for them; preferences have a large impact on what we choose to eat. This is also why successful dieting in the long run requires that we learn to *prefer* healthier foods, not just start eating them. Putting aside the facts that we innately prefer sweetness, and that fatty foods are biologically rewarding, simply having had greater exposure to these foods will eventually have us coming back for just a taste. ·

We Eat What Tastes Good

Notice that the above-mentioned mere exposure experiments in children and adults used foods that we are likely to consume anyway. Foods in mere exposure studies typically include novel cheeses, fruits, tropical juices, and yogurts that all have something in common: they taste pretty good. If researchers didn't choose experimental foods that the children would eat, then they couldn't even do these studies. If you plan to measure amount consumed, then one good research method would be to give participants foods that they will actually consume. Many researchers today teach that we can learn to like healthier foods simply by exposing ourselves to them, and that dieters simply need to be patient while their "taste buds get trained." It is true that we will prefer a flavored tropical drink that we have consumed twenty times compared with another flavored drink that we have consumed only ten times. Unfortunately, the world is not as controlled as a research laboratory. We do not have the luxury of eliminating a lifetime of experiences of eating the foods and flavors we like. Most people have years more experience with sweet-tasting, fatty foods than they do with bitter-tasting, healthier foods. The world's testing trial doesn't involve one flavored drink versus another—it involves an entire cuisine of options. Being patient while our taste buds are trained will invariably take years if we really want to change our diets for life. I don't know many dieters who are that patient!

This doesn't mean your diet is doomed, by any means. It is true that researchers have demonstrated strong positive correlations between preferences and intake in children—as preferences increase, so also does consumption of those preferred foods.[24] In other words, there is strong evidence that children eat the foods they prefer. Yet, although parents provide early feeding experiences to infants, research suggests that the similarities between the later food preferences of parents and those of their children are relatively small.[25] While this may seem counterintuitive, researchers have noted that these findings represent differences in *food* preferences, not *flavor* preferences. In other words, we likely acquire dietary preferences from our parents specifically based on how good the foods taste and smell, not necessarily on what foods the parents eat.

In the next section we will review how we learn about the foods and flavors in our diet through associative processes, society, and culture. This section will provide useful insights into how people can overcome all of this biology, genetics, and mere exposure by explaining how we learn about food and diet—after all, what is learned can be modified! In all, these chapters will bring feeding into context by examining how we learn about the flavors of food and how social-cultural factors influence human feeding.

Notes

1. Hauser, G. J., Chitayat, D., Berbs, L., Braver, D., & Mulbauer, B. (1985). Peculiar odors in newborns and maternal pre-natal ingestion of spicy foods. *European Journal of Pediatrics, 44,* 403.
2. Crystal, S. R., & Bernstein, I. L. (1998). Infant salt preference and mother's morning sickness. *Appetite,* 30 (3), 297-307.
3. Schaal, B., Marlier, L., & Soussignan, R. (2000). Human fetuses learn from their pregnant mother's diet. *Chemical Senses,* 26 (6), 729-737.
4. Mennella, J. A., Johnson, A., & Beauchamp, G. K. (1995). Garlic ingestion by pregnant women alters the odor of amniotic fluid. *Chemical Senses, 20,* 207-209.
5. Hepper, P. G. (1988). Adaptive fetal learning: Prenatal exposure to garlic affects postnatal preferences. *Animal Behavior, 36,* 935-936.
6. Varendi, H., Porter, R. H., & Winberg, J. (2002). The effect of labor on olfactory exposure learning within the first postnatal hour. *Behavioral Neuroscience,* 116 (2), 206-211.
7. Kisilevsky, B. S., Hains, S. M. J., Lee, K., Xie, X., Huang, H., Ye, H. H., Zhang, K., & Wang, Z. (2003). Effects of experience on fetal voice recognition. *Psychological Science,* 14 (3), 220-224.
8. Schaal, B., Marlier, L., & Soussignan, R. (1998). Olfactory function in the human fetus: Evidence from selective neonatal responsiveness to the odor of amniotic fluid. *Behavioral Neuroscience, 112,* 1438-1449.

9. Marlier, L., Schaal, B., & Soussignan, R. (1998). Bottle-fed neonates prefer and odor experienced in utero to an odor experienced postnatally in the feeding context. *Developmental Psychobiology, 33*, 133-45.
10. Mennella, J. A., & Beauchamp, G. K. (1991). Maternal diet alters the sensory qualities of human milk and the nursling's behavior. *Pediatrics, 88*, 737-744.
11. Hepper, P. G. (1996). Fetal memory: Does it exist? What does it do? *Acta Paediatrica, 416* (Sup), 16-20.
12. Blass, E. M., & Camp, C. A. (2001). The ontogeny of face recognition: Eye contact and sweet taste induce face preference in 9- and 12-week-old human infants. *Developmental Psychology, 37* (6), 762-774.
13. Oram, N., Laing, D. G., Freeman, M. H., & Hutchinson, I. (2001). Analysis of taste mixtures by adults and children. *Developmental Psychobiology, 38* (1), 67-77.
14. Pugh, L. C., Milligan, R. A., Frick, K. D., Spatz, D., & Bronner, Y. (2002). Breastfeeding duration, costs, and benefits of a support program for low-income breastfeeding women. *Birth*, 29 (2), 95-100.
15. North, K., Emmett, P., & Noble, S. (2000). Types of drinks consumed by infants at 4 and 8 months of age: Sociodemographic variations. *Journal of Human Nutrition & Dietetics*, 13 (2), 71-82.
16. Mezzacappa, E. S., & Katkin, E. S. (2002). Breast-feeding is associated with reduced perceived stress and negative mood in mothers. *Health Psychology*, 21 (2), 187-191.
17. Gerrish, C. J., & Mennella, J. A. (2000). Short-term influence of breastfeeding on the infants' interaction with the environment. *Developmental Psychobiology*, 36 (1), 40-48.
18. Mennella, J. A., & Beauchamp, G. K. (1996). The human infants' response to vanilla flavors in mother's milk and formula. *Infant behavior and development, 19*, 13-19.
19. Haller, R., Rummel, C., Henneberg, S., Pollmer, U., & Koester, E. P. (1999). The influence of early experience with vanillin on food preference later in life. *Chemical Senses*, 24 (4), 645-647.
20. Mennella, J. A., & Beauchamp, G. K. (2002). Flavor experiences during formula feeding are related to preferences during childhood. *Early Human Development, 68*, 71-82.
21. Liem, D. G., & Mennella, J. A. (2002). Sweet and sour preferences during childhood: Role of early experiences. *Developmental Psychobiology*, 41 (4), 388-395.
22. Birch, L. L., & Marlin, D. W. (1982). I don't like it; I've never tried it: Effects of exposure on two-year-old children's food preferences. *Appetite*, 3 (4), 353-360.
23. Pliner, P. (1982). The effects of mere exposure on liking for edible substances. *Appetite, 3* (3), 283-290.
24. Birch, L. L. (1979). Preschool children's food preferences and consumption patterns. *Journal of Nutrition Education, 11*, 77-80.
25. Birch, L. L. (1980). The relationship between children's food preferences and those of their parents. *Journal of Nutrition Education, 12*, 14-18.

SECTION III: Learning and Diet Acquisition

Chapter 7: Flavor Aversion Learning

Learning is undoubtedly fundamental to the development of controls on food intake.[1] Associative learning plays a central role, such that contextual properties (when and where a food is consumed), sensory properties (color, texture, smell, taste, etc.), and affective properties (positive or negative consequences of consumption) of a food not only can become associated with the food itself, but also can influence how much we like or dislike that food. When animals and humans consume a novel food before or during an aversive event (such as illness or nausea), they subsequently tend to avoid that food. This is referred to as *taste aversion learning*, also called *flavor aversion learning*,[2,3] and it affects primarily the variety of foods in our diets. In a classic study, Garcia and colleagues found that rats preferred to consume a solution of saccharin-flavored water as opposed to tap water. When the researchers later exposed these subjects to gamma radiation (which causes an unconditioned nausea response) while the rats were drinking the saccharin-flavored water, they observed that the rats subsequently avoided this solution.[4] Presumably, saccharin-flavored water became a conditioned cue for nausea, and this phenomenon was termed a conditioned taste aversion.

Aversions can have positive or adverse effects on diet depending on the foods or nutrients for which we acquire aversions. For example, an aversion to foods that are harmful or contain poisons, such as certain types of mushrooms, would be useful. But aversions to other foods or nutrients, such as nutritious vegetables and fruits, would be undesirable. Even the basic tastes that we innately like (i.e., sweet and salty) are just as likely as those we dislike (i.e., sour and bitter) to become aversive when accompanied by a nauseous state;[5] therefore, preferred foods are not exempt from aversion learning. What makes this form of learning unique is that it occurs very rapidly, and it can operate even with long delays between consumption and the onset of illness.[6] It is not uncommon for aversions to be acquired to tastes consumed hours prior to the experience of illness. Long-lasting aversions to *novel* (new) tastes are readily established following only a single taste-illness pairing. Simply stated, conditioned taste aversions are very robust and have been widely demonstrated with little difficulty in animals and humans.

Cue-To-Consequence Learning

Rats, a rodent commonly used in feeding studies, express rather specific aversions following conditioning. In a landmark study, Garcia and colleagues measured associations between conditioned cues (e.g., saccharin or light flash/white noise) and illness caused by radiation exposure or pain produced by shock.[7] They found that saccharin was associated with illness, while audiovisual stimuli (the light flash/white noise stimulus) were associated with shock, despite the fact that saccharin, noise, and light had all been paired equally with both illness and shock. These findings have come to be known as *cue-to-consequence* learning, which generally posits that not all cues are equally well associated with biologically relevant events. Most rodent studies in the literature have confirmed this conclusion: flavor aversions appear to be specific to the consequence following ingestion. Cues that are not ingested (such as visual cues) are not readily associated with illness (or nausea).

For good or bad, these results do not appear to generalize entirely to the cognitively dominated human omnivore. For example, Paul Rozin first noted that humans not only acquire aversions to foods that make them sick (i.e., cause nausea), but also report aversions to foods that are disgusting to them.[8] *Disgust* is defined as "that form of food rejection which is characterized by revulsion at the prospect of oral incorporation of an offensive and contaminating object."[9] Disgust includes even the thought of consumption. We don't have to consume a food, but simply to think of it as disgusting. A recent study showed that 19% of aversions could be classified as *cognitive*—those not caused by a specific taste-illness pairing. Among those reporting cognitive aversions, most attributed the aversion to a disgusting event. Here is one example of a subject's response concerning a disgusting event, as cited in this study: "My little sister got carsick and threw up chicken noodle soup all over me. I haven't eaten chicken noodle soup since—the thought of it makes me ill. I don't like soup in general now, but I liked it before."[10]

While certain foods do appear to disgust us all—especially foods deriving from animals—humans can express disgust and therefore aversion to any number of foods that never actually made them ill. Unlike animals, we readily express aversion to more than just tastes. We don't need to consume a food to acquire an aversion to it; we simply need to think of it as disgusting. Thus, while most human aversions are mediated by taste-illness pairings, human cognition ensures that we will express aversion to more than just these tastes. Just ask my father, who after getting ill while eating in a Burger King as an adolescent, will not eat at any fast-food restaurant today. Decades later, his aversion still persists for more than just the food that made him sick.

Aversions Last a Long Time

Aversion learning is so pronounced that evidence from human studies suggests food aversions can persist for decades. The difficultly in assessing this resistance, though, comes from the procedural nature of measuring such aversions. Aversions are typically measured by allowing a subject to choose between a flavor that was paired with illness and another flavor that was not. This allows the subject to avoid completely the flavor that had made him or her nauseous (by choosing the alternative flavor). Thus, by avoiding the flavor, they never experience an *extinction procedure*—they do not allow repeated exposure to the presumably aversive flavor, even if they could consume it without ill consequence. While an extinction procedure will increase the likelihood that a person will begin to eat a formerly aversive food, it is simply an impractical clinical solution. It would be ethically questionable (at best) for health professionals to force patients to eat foods they do not wish to eat. It could work, but it is not a practical solution.

Many reports have asserted that people not only avoid eating foods that make them ill, but that they also can accurately recall the incident that led to this aversion.[11] English philosopher John Locke noted that a person who eats too much honey might later feel ill merely at the mention of the word.[12] In other words, humans express aversion not only to things they ingest, but also to cognitions about what made them ill, which can make extinguishing an aversion even more challenging. Few people try foods or flavors to which they have acquired aversions, because they also express aversion to the mere thought of those foods. As will be discussed in the final section of this chapter, this has serious implications for limiting the variety of foods we are willing to eat. Still, there appear to be exceptions in regard to whether taste aversions are long-lasting—particularly those acquired during pregnancy.

Food Aversions During Pregnancy

Recent data suggest that aversions acquired during pregnancy may be mediated by taste aversion learning. Pregnancy, which is often characterized by vomiting and nausea, particularly in the first trimester, makes women uniquely prone to aversions. Over 80% of expectant mothers experience nausea and over 50% report some degree of vomiting.[13] One recent study found that 60% of women experience nausea in the same week they report acquiring aversions to foods.[14] These reports strongly indicate that aversions acquired during pregnancy may be mediated by taste-aversion learning.

The most common aversions reported during pregnancy are toward non-alcoholic caffeinated drinks (e.g., teas and coffees), meat, fish, poultry, and eggs.[15] Many theories have been proposed to explain why taste aversions are so common to these foods during pregnancy. The most recent explanation, called *the maternal embryo protection hypothesis*, emphasizes the biological relevance of food aversions for the mother and fetus.[16] This hypothesis states that nausea and vomiting protect the embryo from harmful teratogenic and abortifacient chemicals by physically expelling and subsequently causing avoidance of foods that made the mother ill during pregnancy. Thus, this response (mediated by taste-aversion learning) is meant to protect both the mother and fetus. Like the general population, expectant mothers report having food aversions following only a single food-illness episode even when hours separated the eating of the food and the nauseous experience. This is consistent with a taste-aversion learning explanation.

The supposed cause of food aversions during pregnancy is rather specific. Pregnant women report food aversions following feelings of nausea, but there is no correlation between food aversions and vomiting. Thus, nausea appears to play a particularly important role in the acquisition and expression of food aversions during pregnancy. This has been proposed for the general population and may be characteristic of taste aversions learning in general. For example, research with both animals and humans has shown that feelings of nausea are both sufficient and necessary for the development of flavor aversions.[17,18] Even disgust—thought to cause aversions specifically in humans—produces feelings of nausea. Still, unlike aversions in the general population, aversions acquired during pregnancy don't commonly persist postpartum.[19] Thus, when the pregnancy is over, so is the aversion. One likely explanation is that aversions acquired during pregnancy can be attributed to the pregnancy itself (instead of to specific foods). Thus, once the pregnancy is over, women will consume these foods again, since the pregnancy, not the foods, was viewed as the cause of the nausea.

Still, although nausea is common during pregnancy, expectant mothers acquire aversions to an average of only two foods during a pregnancy, whereas they experience many more than two episodes of nausea on average. This seems counterintuitive at first, since each episode of nausea would be expected to cause an aversion to the food consumed at that time. To explain this, researchers point out that aversions are less likely to occur with foods we are familiar with, especially the foods we eat as part of our preferred diet. This is referred to as *latent inhibition*.

Latent Inhibition

Humans have evolved two known mechanisms for preventing or minimizing aversions to good and safe foods—latent inhibition and neophobia. In terms of eating, *latent inhibition* is the failure to acquire, or slower acquisition of, an aversion. This resistance to acquiring an aversion is a result of previous exposure. It is closely related to mere exposure in that the previous exposure is not reinforced. Simply put, the more mere exposure one has with a food prior to becoming sick after eating it, the less the likelihood that the person will acquire an aversion to the food. Aversions are more likely to develop to novel (or new) foods and slower to develop to familiar ones.[20,21] For example, if you like steak and eat it often, then becoming sick after eating it is not likely to stop you from eating it again. On the other hand, you are much more likely to stop eating steak if you had never tried it before getting sick after eating it.

We want (and find reinforcing) our diets with the sweet, salty, and fatty foods that we like innately. The foods in our diets are those with which we are more familiar, which not only causes us to like them more, but also interferes with efforts to learn to dislike them. In essence, we must overcome a lot of exposure, liking, and neurobiology to learn to dislike the foods from our regular diets. But in a world without supermarkets, fast-food restaurants, and nutrition labels, this system works to our benefit. It motivates us (without learning) to consume safe foods, such as those that taste sweet, and foods that are high in calories, such as fat. In addition (without learning), we eat salty foods, and we need salt to balance out the saltwater in our bodies. Not only does our biology seek the foods that keep us alive, but it also has developed mechanisms to keep us from avoiding these foods if we have found them safe in the past. Since mere exposure increases liking, and therefore the probability that we will eat; latent inhibition ensures that the foods we eat a lot—foods that have been safe and reinforcing in the past—will continue to be consumed, even if they happen to make us sick on one occasion. On the other hand, we will acquire aversions much faster if we become sick after having foods we don't eat as much, including the healthier food options many of us tend not to include in our diets.

In a world without the culinary amenities we enjoy in Western society today, this system ensured that we would eat the foods that were safe and contained needed nutrients, while also ensuring that we would quickly avoid relatively novel foods that make us sick, and could cause death. In sum, the system is nothing less than an innate FDA-approved package label for what is good and nutritious (in terms of calories) for us to eat. Still, we have developed another mechanism for avoiding foods that could make us sick or even kill us, our innate reluctance to eat new foods, called *neophobia*.

Neophobia

While many toxins are readily identifiable by their bitter taste—which we innately dislike—this is not true for all toxins. In order for us to take advantage of learning that a substance is poisonous, it is important that we live after eating it. *Neophobia*—our innate reluctance to consume novel-flavored foods and drinks—is the mechanism that has evolved to cope with this problem. The advantageous logic of such a behavior works like this: if a food is toxic, then cautious sampling may lead to temporary illness rather than death, allowing the animal to live and to avoid that food later.

This phenomenon was first studied in rats, who are notoriously neophobic.[22] So also are children—just ask the millions of parents who find it rather difficult to introduce new foods into a child's diet. You could ask many adults, too—the ones who are reluctant to order new menu items when they visit restaurants, for example. Thus, acquiring aversions to familiar foods is difficult (latent inhibition) and introducing new foods to our diets is also difficult (neophobia). Therefore, the majority of tastes, odors, flavors, and foods we accept as part of our diets are likely to be acquired early in life. What flavors and foods we are willing to eat later in life will depend on a multitude of factors, much of which will be biased by our early feeding experiences.

Aversions Can Limit Diet Variety

Ultimately, aversion learning can limit significantly the ability to shift dieting preferences, thereby limiting the variety of foods we are willing to consume. This is particularly important for clinical populations undergoing aversive therapies. For example, researchers have shown not only that chemotherapy patients form aversions to flavors associated with their treatments,[23] but that these flavors can trigger physical symptoms of nausea even when they are not followed by chemotherapy.[24] Consequently, the symptoms of nausea and vomiting can be elicited in *anticipation* of pharmacological treatments. In an early experiment, Ilene Bernstein showed that children undergoing chemotherapy expressed greater dislike toward and avoidance of a specific food (i.e., a distinctively flavored ice cream) eaten before a clinic visit, when compared with controls.[25] Given the routine nature and necessity for such aversive treatments, these populations are likely at greater risk for limiting diet through taste aversion learning, especially in children.

Still, preferences for foods are much more common than aversions. While all people report preferences for certain foods or flavors in their diets, only a percentage of the general population will report having even a single aversion.[26] This means that the primary means by which we acquire dietary choices is via flavor preference learning. In other words, our dietary choices are mediated most commonly by an active seeking-out of the foods we like, rather than avoidance of the foods we dislike. In the next chapter we will review what is know about this primary mechanism for learning about diet—*flavor reinforcement learning*.

Notes

1.　Davidson, T. L., & Benoit, S. C. (1998). Learning and eating. In O'Donohue, W. T. (Ed.), *Learning and Behavior Therapy* (pp. 498-517). Reno, NV: Prentice Hall.
2.　Capaldi, E. D., Hunter, M. J., & Privitera, G. J. (2004). Odor of taste stimuli in conditioned "taste" aversion learning. *Behavioral Neuroscience*, 118 (6), 1400-1408.
3.　Privitera, G. J., & Capaldi, E. D. (2006). The basic tastants in aversion conditioning: Evidence for sensory preconditioning and not potentiation. *Learning & Behavior*, 34 (4), 355-360.
4.　Garcia, J., Kimeldorf, D. J., & Koelling, R. A. (1955). A conditioned aversion towards saccharin resulting from exposure to gamma radiation. *Science, 122,* 157-158.

5. Nowlis, G. H., Frank, M. E., & Pfaffmann, C. (1980). Specificity of acquired aversions to taste qualities in hamsters and rats. *Journal of Comparative and Physiological Psychology, 94,* 932-942.

6. Garcia, J., Hankins, W. G., & Rusiniak, K. W. (1974). Behavioral regulation of the milieu interne in man and rat. *Science, 185,* 824-831.

7. Garcia, J., & Koelling, R. A. (1966). Relation of cue to consequence in avoidance learning. *Psychonomic Science,* 4 (3), 123-124.

8. Rozin P. (1986). One-trial acquired likes and dislikes in humans: Disgust as a US, food predominance, and negative learning predominance. *Learning and Motivation, 17,* 180-189.

9. Rozin, P., & Fallon, A. E. (1987). A perspective on disgust (cited on pp. 24). *Psychological Review, 94,* 23-41.

10. Batsell, W. R. Jr., & Brown, A. S. (1998). Human flavor aversion learning: A comparison of traditional aversions and cognitive aversions (cited in Table 2, pp. 389). *Learning and Motivation, 29,* 383-396.

11. Logue, A. W., Ophir, I., & Strauss, K. E. (1981). The acquisition of taste aversion in humans. *Behavior Research and Therapy, 19,* 319-333.

12. Chance, P. (1999). *Learning and Behavior* (4th ed., cited on pp. 119). Pacific Grove, CA: Brooks/Cole Publishing Company.

13. Tierson, F. D., Olsen, C. L., & Hook, E. B. (1986). Nausea and vomiting of pregnancy and association with pregnancy outcome. *American Journal of Obstetrics and Gynecology, 155,* 1017-1022.

14. Bayley, T. M., Dye, L., Jones, S., DeBono, M., & Hill, A. J. (2002). Food cravings and aversions during pregnancy: Relationships with nausea and vomiting. *Appetite, 38,* 45-51.

15. Flaxman, S. M., & Sherman, P. W. (2000). Morning sickness: Mechanism for protecting mother and embryo. *Quarterly Review of Biology, 75,* 113-148.

16. Profet, M. (1995). *Protecting your baby-to-be: Preventing birth defects in the first trimester.* New York: Addison-Wesley Publishing.

17. Garcia, J. (1989). Food for Tolman: Cognition and cathexis in concert. In T. Archer & L. G. Nelson (Eds.), *Aversion, Avoidance, and Anxiety* (pp. 45-85). Hillsdale, NJ: Erlbaum.

18. Pelchat, M. L., & Rozin, P. (1982). The special role of nausea in the acquisition of food dislikes in humans. *Appetite, 3,* 341-351.

19. Worthington-Roberts, B., Little, R. E., Lambert, M. D., & Wu, R. (1989). Dietary cravings and aversions in the postpartum period. *Journal of the American Dietetic Association, 89,* 647-651.

20. Revusky, S. H., & Bedarf, E. W. (1967). Association of illness with prior ingestion of novel foods. *Science, 155,* 219-220.

21. Kalat, J. W., & Rozin, P. (1973). "Learned safety" as a mechanism in long-delay taste aversion learning in rats. *Journal of Comparative and Physiological Psychology, 83,* 198-207.

22. Rozin, P., & Kalat, J. W. (1971). Specific hungers and poison avoidance as adaptive specializations of learning. *Psychological Review, 78,* 459-486.

23. Carey, M. P., & Burish, T. G. (1988). Etiology and treatment of the psychological side effects associated with cancer chemotherapy: A critical review and discussion. *Psychological Bulletin, 104,* 307-325.

24. Bovbjerg, D. H., Redd, W. H., Jacobsen, P. B., Manne, S. L., Taylor, K. L., Surbone, A., Crown, J. P., Norton, L., Gilewski, T. A., Hudis, C. A., Reichman, B. S.,

Kaufman, R. J., Currie, V. E., & Hakes, T. B. (1992). An experimental analysis of classically conditioned nausea during cancer chemotherapy. *Psychosomatic Medicine, 54*, 623-637.

25. Bernstein, I. L. (1978). Learned taste aversions in children receiving chemotherapy. *Science, 200*, 1302-1303.

26. Garb, J. L., & Stunkard, A. J. (1974). Taste aversions in man. *American Journal of Psychiatry, 131*, 1204-1207.

Chapter 8: Flavor Reinforcement Learning

Most food preferences are produced by experience, through either mere exposure or *flavor reinforcement* (flavor-taste and flavor nutrient-learning). We undoubtedly learn a great deal from the consequences of our actions, and this includes the consequences of what we choose to eat. This is not meant to minimize the fact that our dietary choices are biased by our biology—such as our innate preference for sweet-tasting foods. In fact, it is these very biases that primarily mediate how we learn about the rich array of flavors in our diets—we learn to like most foods by tasting them.[1] Both animals and humans learn about the flavors associated with the tastes and nutrients they consume. Although humans may not be able to count the calories they consume, both animals and humans can learn to like them.

This chapter will review what we know about the processes by which we acquire preferences for foods. There are four known ways to increase liking: mere exposure (the subject of an earlier chapter), the medicine effect, flavor-taste learning, and flavor-nutrient learning. These four, all forms of learning, are more straightforward and practical than you may think. The reality is that unless we like the foods we eat, we will eventually stop eating them. There are few exceptions to this rule—we eat what we like, for good or bad.

The Medicine Effect

Foods and flavors associated with recovery from illness come to be liked. This effect is referred to as the *medicine effect* and has been readily demonstrated in rats.[2] For example, rats will acquire and express an aversion to a flavor consumed 30 minutes prior to or following an injection of lithium chloride (an unconditioned cue for nausea). But, if another flavor is presented 75 minutes following the injection—a time course when rats begin to recover from the effects of this emetic drug—rats increase consumption of the flavor.[3] In other words, they express a preference for the flavor associated with recovery from illness. Unfortunately, while the medicine effect is a rather robust phenomenon in rats, it is not as robust in humans.[4]

Still, the medicine effect has undoubtedly contributed to our evolutionary success. For example, some of the most bitter-tasting plants in nature not only contain nutrients, they also provide valuable medicines. Thus, in order for humans to tolerate the bitterness of these medicines—such as the very bitter sap in opium poppy—they had to adopt ways of learning to overcome (rather, to like) the tastes of these plants. By doing so, humans were able to develop a strategy that uses a basic *law of effect*: a behavior (such as consuming bitter-tasting plants) followed by positive consequences (such as recuperation from illness) will increase the probability of the behavior, and therefore the probability of consuming these medicinal plants again when seeking to recover from illness. This is a simple and very effective biological strategy—behave in the world to seek positive consequences and avoid negative ones. How does our biology accomplish this? It shifts our preferences (i.e., our liking) toward those things that produce positive consequences, even if that requires liking the bitter taste of medicinal plants.

Not that this form of learning is clinically applicable though—I highly discourage people from getting sick simply so that they can increase liking for flavors and foods they consume during recovery. Regardless, preferences resulting from recovery from illness account for very few of the preferences expressed in the general population. The development of most food likes is instead primarily acquired through two alternative processes: flavor-taste and flavor-nutrient learning.

Flavor-Taste Learning

A common method used to increase liking for a flavor is to pair it with an already liked taste. This strategy is referred to as *flavor-taste learning*. Recall that we acquire preferences primarily toward the flavors in our diet, not the foods per se. This makes flavor-taste learning advantageous since it shifts preferences to specific flavors in our diets. By association with a preferred taste (such as the taste of sweet), a less-liked or non-preferred flavor (such as an odor) will subsequently become more liked even when it is no longer paired with the preferred taste.

For this form of preference learning to work, one taste must be innately liked (such as salty and sweet). The innately liked taste does not need to be nutritious—it just needs to taste good. Studies in rats and humans have shown that even nutritionally deplete solutions that taste good can increase liking to arbitrary flavors. For example, saccharin and Equal sweetener contain no calories, but they taste sweet. In one study, rats received two arbitrary flavors (cinnamon and wintergreen). One flavor was mixed with a higher concentration of saccharin (a taste); the other with a lower concentration. After several exposures to these sweetened flavors, the rats were given a choice between unsweetened cinnamon and wintergreen. This test showed that subjects consumed significantly more of the flavor that had been mixed with the higher concentration of saccharin, even though this flavor was no longer sweetened.[5] Thus, even though saccharin is a nutritionally useless taste, it still increased preferences for a less-preferred flavor that was mixed with it. This means that without consuming calories, you can increase preference for healthier foods. There are numerous studies using both humans and animals that show this process to be effective at increasing liking and subsequent preference for flavors that were initially not liked at all. For example, human studies have shown that undergraduates receiving several exposures to unfamiliar sweetened and unsweetened teas express an increased preference for the flavor of the tea that had been sweetened, even when it is no longer sweetened.[6]

Still, dieters are ultimately interested in increasing their liking for nutritious foods, such as vegetables and fruits, not teas. As it turns out, flavor-taste reinforcement can increase liking for flavors that are disliked, such as those bitter-tasting vegetables and sour-tasting fruits. For example, our research has shown that mixing broccoli and cauliflower with sugar can increase pleasantness ratings for these vegetables in college students.[7] In one study, we gave some college student's sweetened broccoli and unsweetened cauliflower; others received sweetened cauliflower and unsweetened broccoli. When later tested with unsweetened broccoli and cauliflower, students rated as more pleasant the vegetable that had been given to them earlier as sweetened, as opposed to the vegetable they had been given earlier as unsweetened. In a second experiment, we showed this effect with sour-tasting fruits in children. Unsweetened grapefruit juice has a very sour taste that makes it unpalatable to many children and adults. Mixing grapefruit juice with high concentrations of sweet-tasting sucrose increased liking for the sour taste of grapefruit juice in children (two to five years old). In fact, not only did preference ratings increase for unsweetened grapefruit juice immediately following the flavor-taste pairings, but also a follow-up test two weeks later showed that the children still reported liking unsweetened grapefruit juice. This is consistent with previously published reports indicating that flavor-taste associations can provide one mechanism for liking.

Unfortunately, despite the effectiveness of this learning strategy, only about one-third of parents report that they use this method to shift children's food preferences.[8] One concern for parents may be with the use of sugars and sweeteners to increase liking. If this is a concern, parents should be aware of two important characteristics of this method for learning. First, preferences are thought to shift permanently. In most cases, sweetening foods for only a few weeks can cause permanent shifts in liking, even after the sweetener is no longer added. It is a temporary and relatively short-term intervention that has long-term results. Second, the sweeteners do not need to contain calories; they simply need to taste sweet. You may have noticed that the sugar mixed with the vegetables and the sucrose mixed with the grapefruit juice not only tasted good (flavor-taste learning), but also contained calories (flavor-nutrient learning). As implied by flavor-nutrient learning (which we will discuss next), pairing flavors with nutrients in the form of calories can also increase preferences.

It is well known that foods that taste good also contain lots of calories. As a result, it is often difficult to distinguish between flavor-taste and flavor-nutrient learning. Say you have a sweet-tasting, calorie-containing, apple-flavored fruit drink—does the sweet taste (flavor-taste) or the calories (flavor-nutrient) increase liking for the apple-flavored drink? The answer is both, although, as you will learn, our liking for calories tends to be stronger than our liking for tastes. Experimentally, one way to distinguish between these forms of learning is to recognize that flavor-taste learning is limited by delay. The delay between the time the disliked flavor and the liked taste are consumed must be less than nine seconds for flavor-taste learning to be effective at increasing preference.[9] Flavor-taste preferences are most enhanced when a non-preferred flavor is mixed with a taste that the person likes—such as mixing vegetables and fruits with sugars. Separating the liked taste from the disliked taste significantly decreases how much flavor-taste preference is enhanced. Flavor-nutrient learning is not limited by such delays; this is reviewed in the next section.

Flavor-Nutrient Learning

Another common method used to increase liking for a flavor is to pair it with nutrients (measured in calories). Among the nutrients we consume, the highest caloric nutrient—and likely the most reinforcing—is dietary fat. Consumption of this nutrient alone will have a significant impact on the nutritional quality of our diets and on short- and long-term weight gain. Children who report preferences for flavors or foods that are high in fat tend to weigh more and consume more calories than those who report fewer preferences for these foods.[10] Unfortunately, many of the volatile substances that make foods flavorful are fat-soluble; thus, high-fat foods tend to taste great.[11] Still, learning to prefer all of the flavors associated with these calories doesn't require the dieter to continue consuming these fats. After learning takes place, we could reduce or eliminate the fats and still like (even prefer) the flavor of our diets.

This strategy is referred to as *flavor-nutrient learning*. What makes this form of learning particularly interesting is that it seems to contradict a major theme in this book—that humans cannot feel their calories. Apparently, though, this is specific to feelings of hunger and fullness. Our biology is such that it has multiple systems in place to monitor, store, and use calories. Yet, we judge fullness and hunger—our behavioral strategy for systematically seeking and ingesting an appropriate number of calories—based on alternative factors that *infer* how many calories we consume. As it turns out, our "intuitive biology" developed another means of ensuring that we will consume those calories, regardless of whether they satiate us: we learn to like them. We eat what we like; therefore, liking high-calorie foods will biologically and behaviorally ensure that we attend to, seek, and consume those calories.

For this form of preference learning to work, one flavor must have been previously associated with calories. But again, what tastes good also tends to be high in calories. For example, many people do not initially like the taste of coffee. However, with the addition of sugars (sweet taste + calories) and high-fat creamers (more calories), the flavor of coffee becomes more acceptable (or palatable) to the point where it can later be consumed black (i.e., without the sugars and creamers). Flavor-taste and flavor-nutrient learning contribute simultaneously to many of our learned preferences. The key distinction appears to be the delay in learning; flavor-nutrient preferences are expressed even if subjects receive calories hours after consuming a flavor.[12]

Since flavor-taste learning does not occur at appreciable delays (more than nine seconds), researchers have studied flavor-nutrient learning by including a significant delay between the presentation of an arbitrary flavor and the presentation of nutrients. Animal studies demonstrate flavor-nutrient preferences in rats to flavors presented thirty minutes prior to the presentation of a variety of caloric reinforcers including dextrose, polycose, and a high-fat wet mash.[13] Regardless of what reinforcer was used, flavor-nutrient preferences were expressed. The thirty-minute delay between flavor and nutrient presentations would be too long for flavor-taste preferences to account for this learning. Studies such as these have been taken as evidence that flavor-nutrient learning is distinct from flavor-taste learning.

Another method for distinguishing between flavor-taste and flavor-nutrient learning takes advantage of the fact that certain tastes are innately liked or disliked, as discussed in chapter 5. For example, animal researchers have mixed various Kool-Aid flavors with liked tastes (corn oil or sucrose) and disliked tastes (ethanol) that all contained the same number of calories.[14] They found that all subjects expressed similar preferences for the Kool-Aid flavors regardless of whether they were mixed with the liked taste (i.e., corn oil or sucrose) or disliked taste (i.e., ethanol). If flavor-taste learning were involved, we would expect preferences to differ between subjects receiving a *flavor-liked taste* pairing versus a *flavor-disliked taste* pairing. Instead, all subjects formed similar preferences, which can be fully attributed to the equal number of calories in each flavor-taste mixture. This also suggests that flavor-nutrient learning can override or interfere with flavor-taste learning, because of the introduction of calories.

This has also been shown in our human studies. In one study, undergraduate students received orange- or banana-flavored, bitter-tasting cream cheese crackers with either low- or high-fat cream cheeses.[15] Based on flavor-taste learning, subjects should express low pleasantness ratings for a bitter-tasting cream cheese cracker. Based on flavor nutrient learning, subjects should express greater pleasantness ratings for the high-fat (higher-calorie) cream cheese cracker than its low-fat alternative. Indeed, results showed that the flavors associated with high-fat cream cheeses were rated as more pleasant than flavors associated with low-fat cream cheeses, even though all cream cheese crackers tasted bitter (a disliked taste). Similar to the animal studies, we showed that flavor-nutrient learning could override or interfere with flavor-taste learning. Animals and humans essentially like high-calorie flavors (flavor-nutrient learning) more than flavors that just taste great (flavor-taste learning)—although both strategies will increase liking for less-preferred flavors.

Flavor-nutrient learning is likely responsible for the human fat preference as well. While humans are poor at estimating caloric intake, let alone differences in caloric density, there are ways of cheating, so to speak. Fat has a lot of calories—nine per gram, compared with four calories per gram for protein and carbohydrates. Thus, one likely mechanism that produces our innate preference for the taste of fat is its reliable association with a high-density load of calories. Therefore, it is not necessary to compute or "feel" calories, simply to learn what tastes and flavors are associated with all of those calories and make them liked—since we eat what we like, this ensures that we will eat foods high in calories. Still, reinforcing people with lots of calories to get them to like less-preferred foods does not always work—a phenomenon most commonly referred to as the *dessert effect*.

Dessert and Contrast Effects

A recent study with schoolchildren found that (among other behavioral strategies) providing a dessert reward resulted in greater acceptance of a novel food.[16] This may seem obvious, since many parents use dessert as a means of motivating children to consume healthier foods in a meal. The problem is that this strategy is short-term and many times produces the opposite effect we desire—children learn to like the dessert more, not the healthier foods in the meal. Indeed, while this study did demonstrate increased *acceptance* of the novel foods, it is likely (depending on how rewarding the dessert was to the children) these children would not have reported that the novel foods were more *liked*. In fact, only 7% of parents report that rewarding their children for eating a food increased liking for that food.[17]

A meal is complex in that many foods and flavors are consumed in a single sitting. This means that there is a lot of flavor-taste and flavor-nutrient learning going on every time we sit down to eat a meal. Presumably, the healthier foods on your plate, such as the sour-tasting fruits, are associated with the more-preferred foods, such as the high-fat French fries or steak you are eating at the meal. Each time you have a meal, you are engaging in a flavorful learning experience. The more you eat vegetables, fruits, and other healthier, less-preferred food options in the same meal as your more-preferred foods, the more you set the stage for learning to prefer these healthier foods via flavor-taste and flavor-nutrient learning.

But what flavors or foods become associated with the calories we consume in the same meal (flavor-nutrient learning)? As it turns out, the calories are associated with whatever we consume last—which many times means that the high-fat, high-calorie, sweet-tasting dessert gets all the credit for the calories we consume. This has important implications for flavor reinforcement learning because—as mentioned in the previous section—flavor-nutrient learning can override what we learn from flavor-taste associations. We may not be able to count calories very well, but learning about flavors associated with calories (flavor-nutrient learning) appears to control what we like more than the flavors associated with other liked tastes (flavor-taste learning). This means (in theory) that the dessert-calories association can overshadow much of the flavor-taste learning that took place in that meal.

This effect was first demonstrated in rats. Capaldi and colleagues, for example, gave two groups of rats two meals (rice and potatoes).[18] One group received rice followed by a sweet-tasting dessert (sucrose) and potatoes followed by nothing; the other group received potatoes followed by dessert and rice followed by nothing. Remarkably, in a preference test between rice and potatoes side by side, rats in both groups expressed a preference (i.e., showed greater consumption) for the meal associated with nothing. Since the dessert followed the meal by five minutes, flavor-taste learning couldn't have accounted for the preferences—remember that this learning is not effective with delays greater than nine seconds. Also, these findings have since been replicated.[19]

To explain these results, researchers note that the higher-concentrated reinforcer is so liked that rats suppress consumption of the meal in anticipation of the highly reinforcing dessert—a phenomenon termed *anticipatory negative contrast*.[20] These contrast effects may account for the dessert effect in that potato consumption may have been reduced when followed by sucrose, because rats were anticipating the more preferred sucrose reinforcer. As I would often say as a child, "Gotta save room for dessert!" Essentially, if the dessert is very reinforcing and you know it's coming, then you will reduce consumption of the meal, essentially to save room for that tasty treat. Still, this explanation must be taken with caution since reduced consumption doesn't necessarily mean reduced liking. In fact, decreased consumption and increased liking can occur simultaneously. Therefore, another explanation has been proposed, which also accounts for the dessert effect. This explanation is based on the fact that our cells, which need the calories we consume, don't start actually receiving them until about thirty to forty-five minutes following consumption.

The Postingestive Consequences of Consumption

As part of digestion, the foods we consume have a relatively long way to travel after we ingest them. When food is consumed, it is broken down and digested. It passes through the stomach, pylorus, and duodenum before ever being absorbed into the body. This process takes time, and until the nutrients we consume are absorbed into the body, our cells can't use the energy. Thus, it is not until this absorptive phase, about thirty to forty-five minutes after we begin a meal, that we are experiencing the positive postingestive consequences of consumption. Since the nutrients we consume are not used until our cells begin receiving the energy, then what gets associated with all those calories? While studies have shown that foods consumed earlier in the meal may acquire some flavor-nutrient learning, the overwhelming consensus is that preferences are increased most for the flavors or foods most closely associated (in time) with the nutritional consequences of consumption.[21] In other words, liking for the flavor of the *last* food you eat is increased the most as a result of consuming calories in the meal. In many cases this means, unfortunately, that you increase liking most for the sweet, fatty taste of the dessert and not the healthier foods you consumed earlier.

Collectively, the delayed use of calories will increase preference for the dessert and contrast effects will decrease consumption of the less-preferred foods in the meal—the opposite of what any good-intentioned parent had in mind. Therefore, rewarding a child for eating a disliked food by providing a dessert at the end of a meal is generally going to be ineffective at increasing preferences for anything but the reward itself. It won't necessarily decrease liking for the foods in the meal, but it won't increase liking either. Still, as a meal progress we get fuller, and hunger also affects how much we like the foods we eat. Therefore, it is important to consider how hunger before a meal can affect preferences for the foods we consume in that meal.

Deprivation and Liking

In general, animal studies have shown that foods consumed when hungry are preferred more than foods consumed when satiated or full.[22] Animal studies also indicate that the greater the degree of deprivation, the greater our preferences are for the foods we consume, even when these foods are consumed later when we are satiated.[23] Capaldi and colleagues, for example, gave rats a flavored wet mash (which rats like to eat) under different combinations of deprivation. Subjects consumed these foods for a period of days and were then tested for a preference to the flavor they had consumed while deprived. Researchers found that the highly deprived rats in all groups expressed a preference for the flavored wet mash compared with subjects who were relatively less deprived, regardless of whether subjects were satiated prior to testing for preferences. In other words, the rats continued to prefer the flavor of the foods they had consumed while deprived, even when they were satiated. This is similar to my experience with eating MREs (chapter 1). I ate these meals often during training exercises under high deprivation, and later found myself preferring these meals even when my deprivation had passed.

One caveat, though, is that the foods used in these studies were unsweetened. When sweetened foods are used under similar conditions, for some reason rats express the opposite preferences. They prefer the flavor consumed under low deprivation (satiety) to the flavor consumed under high deprivation (hunger).[24] While researchers have suggested that there is something aversive or unpleasant about consuming sweetened foods when highly food deprived,[25] this effect does not appear to generalize entirely to human preferences. After all, try to convince the millions of people who pour sugar on their cereals or eat sweet-ened fruits in the morning that sweetness doesn't taste good when food de-prived. Since our longest fast (and greatest deprivation) tends to be between dinner and breakfast, people should not be expected to choose sweetened foods for breakfast, but they often do.

A study with undergraduate students showed that changes in deprivation in-deed have no effect on preferences for sweetness.[26] Instead, they showed that increased deprivation was actually associated with increased liking for sweet-ness in many subjects. Regardless of whether students were satiated or deprived, they expressed strong hedonic (liking) responses for sweetness. Of course, as undergraduates, all students likely had significant exposure to sweet-tasting so-lutions (mere exposure learning), which may have contributed to these results. Still, a more recent study showed that healthy university students—after 30 minutes of exercise, which presumably put subjects into a relatively deprived state—showed increased preference ratings for sucrose, glucose, stevioside, D-sorbitol, and erythritol, but not for saccharin.[27] All of these substances taste sweet and were preferred regardless of deprivation. This clearly indicates that taste preferences for many sweet substances does not change, and can actually be increased with greater deprivation in humans. It is interesting to note, though, that saccharin does not contain calories and was the only sweet taste not pre-ferred more following exercise. This suggests that humans judge liking under deprivation based on the caloric value of the sweet-tasting solution and not just the taste per se.

In all, this research implies that the foods we consume while deprived are primarily associated with the calories we consume (flavor-nutrient learning), more so than the taste of the food (flavor-taste learning). Since the calories we consume when highly food deprived would be more rewarding—since our cells are in greater need of energy—this would explain why we continue to like the flavor of these foods later, when satiated. After all, the more deprived we are, the more our cells need that energy—it is no wonder, therefore, that we express a greater need for calories (and liking for the flavors associated with them) over what tastes good, especially when calorie-deprived.

Short-Term Interventions With Long-Term Results

While flavor reinforcement learning in animals is evident following as few as two to four pairings,[28] learning in humans takes a bit longer—usually a few weeks at most. Without any further reinforcement, preferences will persist to the flavors previously associated with reinforcement. These are short-term strategies that produce long-term results. The results are long-term because flavor rein-forcement learning is a sensory phenomenon—preferences for the sensory com-ponents of foods increase as a result of learning. This means that we learn to like the flavors of the foods associated with calories (flavor-nutrient learning) or other liked tastes (flavor-taste learning). We don't simply associate these flavors with reinforcement; we learn to like them even without further reinforcement—referred to as a transfer of affect.

A *transfer of affect* means that the liking for sweetened foods, for example, will shift from the sweet taste to the odors and flavors of foods mixed with them. Even more, humans also report a *transfer of sensation*—human subjects not only like a sweetened flavor more, they also report that it tastes sweet even when the sugar is removed! For example, Stevenson and colleagues examined how repeated pairings of novel odors with sweet and sour tastes alter human perception of an odor presented alone.[29,30,31] Astonishingly, these studies showed that odors mixed with sucrose (sweet-tasting) were rated as smelling sweeter when tested unsweetened; odors mixed with citric acid (sour-tasting) were rated as smelling more sour when tested without the citric acid mixture. Therefore, not only is it likely that you will prefer foods mixed with sweet tastes and dislike foods mixed with sour tastes—you will actually experience them as tasting sweeter or sourer even without the added taste mixtures.

In all, flavor reinforcement preferences are long-term—both in terms of liking and sensory perception. After only a few pairings, you will like and prefer originally disliked or non-preferred foods without the added calories or associations with good tastes. To date, there is no evidence that preferences following flavor reinforcement learning will ever cease, unless you specifically acquire an aversion to these same flavors or foods. In our research, we sweetened broccoli and cauliflower to make them more palatable. After a few pairings, subjects continued to prefer and like the bitter-tasting vegetables without the added sweetener. The children who were given sweetened grapefruit juice also needed only a few weeks of drinking this sweetened juice before they also learned to like the sour taste of grapefruit juice without the added sweetener. Adding fat to cream cheese crackers also increased liking for bitterness in only three sittings. In all, liking for these tastes and flavors persisted even without further reinforcement. We learn to like the flavors and tastes of foods that we never would have consumed or liked before. This preference is long-term—without any further reinforcement, these vegetables, fruits, and cheeses will taste great and be more preferred.

In terms of healthy eating, vegetables and fruits contain few calories, but are highly nutritious. Learning to like them is a key component to including them in our diets long-term. This is because we eat what we like in the long-term. Also, learning to like them means we will like eating fewer calories. For example, recall that feeling full does not appear to be directly related to how many calories we consume. Instead, fullness is determined by factors such as what types of foods (not drinks) we consume, our experiences with them, and how we think of them. Based on the principles reviewed in this book, consuming these lower-calorie foods with higher-calorie preferred options for only a few weeks will make us feel fuller with fewer calories, and increase how much we like those lower-calorie foods as well.

Ultimately, the most successful way to diet long-term would be to learn to like a lower-calorie diet, whether that means eating less of the high-calorie foods, or eating more of the lower-calorie foods, or both. While these strategies may seem too simple, this is all the more reason to use them for improving the health of your diet. In fact, you already are using these strategies every time you put salt on your French fries and steak, eat a dessert at the end of a meal, eat a meal following a long fast, or eat high-fat, high-sugar brownies, ice creams, cookies, cakes, or chips for a snack. Every day we engage in a flavorful learning experience, but most of what we learn actually increases our preferences for the very foods we are trying to avoid—foods that in many cases don't even make us feel full. In all, flavor reinforcement learning accounts for the majority of the preferences we express in our diets—for good and bad.

Notes

1. Birch, L. L., McPhee, L., Shoba, B. C., Pirok, E., & Steinberg, L. (1987). What kind of exposure reduces children's food neophobia? *Appetite, 9*, 171-178.
2. Green, K. F., & Garcia, J. (1971). Recuperation from illness: Flavor enhancement in rats. *Science, 193*, 749-759.
3. Barker, L. M., & Weaver, C. A. III (1991). Conditioning flavor preferences in rats: Dissecting the "medicine effect". *Learning and Motivation, 22*, 311-328.
4. Pliner, P, Rozin, P., Cooper, M., & Woody, G. (1985). Role of specific postingestive effects and medicinal context in the acquisition of liking for tastes. *Appetite, 6*, 243-252.
5. Holman, E. W. (1975). Immediate and delayed reinforcers for flavor preferences in rats. *Animal Learning & Behavior, 6*, 91-100.
6. Zellner, D. A., Rozin, P., Aron, M., & Kulish, D. (1983). Conditioned enhancement of humans' liking for flavors paired with sweetness. *Learning and Motivation, 14*, 338-350.
7. Capaldi, E. D., & Privitera, G. J. (in press). Decreasing dislike for sour and bitter in children and adults. *Appetite.*
8. Casey, R., & Rozin, P. (1989). Changing children's food preferences: Parents' opinions. *Appetite, 12*, 171-182.
9. Lyn, S. A., & Capaldi, E. D. (1994). Robust conditioned flavor preferences with a sensory preconditioning procedure. *Psychonomic Bulletin & Review*, 1 (4), 491-493.
10. Fisher, J. A., & Birch, L. L. (1995). Fat preferences and fat consumption of 3- to 5-year-old children are related to parental adiposity. *Journal of the American Dietetic Association, 95*, 759-764.
11. Birch, L. L. (1992). Children's preferences for high-fat foods. *Nutrition Reviews, 50*, 249-255.
12. Capaldi, E. D., & Sheffer, J. D. (1992). Contrast and reinforcement in consumption. *Learning and Motivation, 23*, 63-79.
13. Capaldi, E. D., Campbell, D. H., Sheffer, J. D., & Bradford, J. P. (1987). Conditioned flavor preferences based on delayed caloric consequences. *Journal of Experimental Psychology: Animal Behavior Processes, 13*, 150-155.
14. Mehiel, R., & Bolles, R. C. (1988). Learned flavor preferences based on calories are independent of initial hedonic value. *Animal Learning & Behavior, 16*, 383-387.
15. Capaldi, E. D., & Privitera, G. J. (in press). Flavor-nutrient learning independent of flavor-taste learning with college students. *Appetite.*

16. Hendy, H. M. (1999). Comparison of five teacher actions to encourage children's new food acceptance. *Annals of Behavioral Medicine*, 21 (1), 20-26.
17. Casey, R. & Rozin, P. (1989). Changing children's food preferences: Parents opinions. *Appetite, 12*, 171-182.
18. Capaldi, E. D., Campbell, D. H., Sheffer, J. D., & Bradford, J. P. (1987). Nonreinforcing effects of giving "desserts" in rats. *Appetite, 9*, 99-112.
19. Capaldi, E. D., Sheffer, J. D., & Pulley, R. J. (1989). Contrast effects in flavor preference learning. *Quarterly Journal of Experimental Psychology*, 41B (3), 307-232.
20. Flaherty, C. F., & Checke, S. (1982). Anticipation of incentive gain. *Animal Learning and Behavior, 10*, 177-182.
21. Elizalde, G., & Sclafani, A. (1988). Starch-based conditioned flavor preferences in rats: Influence of taste, calories, and CS-US delay. *Appetite, 11*, 179-200.
22. Revusky, S. H., Smith, M. H., Jr., & Chalmers, D. V. (1971). Flavor preferences: Effects of ingestion-contingent intravenous saline or glucose. *Physiology & Behavior, 6*, 341-343.
23. Capaldi, E. D., Sheffer, J. D., & Owens, J. (1991). Food deprivation and conditioned flavor preferences based on sweetened and unsweetened foods. *Animal Learning and Behavior, 19*, 361-368.
24. Capaldi, E. D., & Myers, D. E. (1982). Taste preferences as a function of food deprivation during original taste exposure. *Animal Learning and Behavior, 10*, 211-219.
25. Capaldi, E. D. (1996). Conditioned food preferences. In E. D. Capaldi (ed.), *Why We Eat What We Eat: The Psychology of Eating* (pp. 53-82). Washington, D.C.: American Psychological Association.
26. Looy, H., & Weingarten, H. P. (1991). Effects of metabolic state on sweet taste reactivity in humans depend on underlying hedonic response profile. *Chemical Senses*, 16 (2), 123-130.
27. Horio, T. (2004). Effect of physical exercise on human preference for solutions of various sweet substances. *Perceptual and Motor Skills, 99*, 1061-1070.
28. Mehiel, R., & Bolles, R. C. (1988). Learned flavor preferences based on calories are independent of initial hedonic value. *Animal Learning & Behavior, 16*, 383-387.
29. Stevenson, R. J., Prescott, J., & Boakes, R. A. (1995). The acquisition of taste properties by odors. *Learning & Motivation, 26*, 433-455.
30. Stevenson, R. J., Boakes, R. A., & Prescott, J. (1998). Changes in odor sweetness resulting from implicit learning of a simultaneous odor–sweetness association: an example of learned synesthesia. *Learning & Motivation, 29*, 113-132.
31. Stevenson, R. J., Boakes, R. A., & Wilson, J. P. (2000). Resistance to extinction of conditioned odor perceptions: evaluative conditioning is not unique. *Journal of Experimental Psychology: Learning, Memory, & Cognition, 26*, 423-440.

Chapter 9: Sociocultural Factors in Eating

I have been to a few fine restaurants over the years and have found myself asking this question: why is it that the more money I spend on a cuisine, the less food I get on my plate? What is unique about this question (and you may have the same impression) is that it can be asked only if I hold some expectation of what a portion size should be. Most people have some expectation of what is an appropriate portion of food. Even without the pains of fullness, many of us "feel" as if we have eaten too much; or, without necessarily "feeling" hungry, we still desire more food based primarily on how much was in front of us. Of course, these expectations are in part the product of what we have learned through culture and society.

By now it is quite clear that learned factors affect our diets more than just the calories we consume. Biological cues for hunger, satiety, liking, and disliking can all be seemingly overridden by these learned cues, which are acquired through experience, exposure, culture, and society. Thus far, though, we have primarily discussed learning about diet in terms of consuming flavors, tastes, and nutrients. But even without the physical experience of consumption, we still learn a great deal about diet and preferences through society and culture. For example, children will learn to like foods they consume while engaging in a friendly context, such as when they have a positive interaction with a friendly adult.[1] These preferences are mediated by a positive social context, not by the eating per se. Consider another context: say, you want your kids to eat their vegetables. Well, one way to do this is to force them to eat. Many parents will have their children sit at the table until they have "cleaned their plates." The effect of this is actually negative. While children will eventually clean their plates, they learn to dislike the foods as a result because eating them was associated with a negative, coercive context. Thus, by doing this, parents produce greater disliking for the very foods they want their children to like.[2,3] This is another example of how norms for eating can facilitate and/or interfere with the acquisition of healthy diets. We can learn a lot about food through society and culture.

Social and cultural interactions (referred to as *sociocultural*) play a major role in facilitating food likes and dislikes, which ultimately affect diet acquisition. Before the advent of the Food and Drug Administration, the Office of the Surgeon General, or nutritional labels, food selection was presumably much more stressful. Social and cultural norms for meal patterns and dieting were undoubtedly aimed at helping early humans guide their dieting choices toward a stereotyped pattern of eating certain foods known to be good or safe. Establishing such norms would likely reduce the time, energy, and risk associated with diet acquisition. Therefore, it should not be surprising that sociocultural norms, attitudes, beliefs, values, habits, perceptions, etc. all impact our food choices, especially early in life.

Society, Culture, and the Family Paradox

To a large extent, it is through early learning about social and cultural norms that we find out about appropriate portion size, number of meals to consume daily, snacking, and when to eat which foods. When I was a young boy, my Italian family showed me that food was something of which you ate a lot. I could have seconds, thirds, and fourths if I wanted (portion size was essentially unlimited). This may explain why I always seemed to feel cheated by the modest portion sizes served at many fine, expensive restaurants. In the modern world, humans simply cannot escape the cultural and social influences affecting the choices they make, including those concerning their diets.

Cultural factors affect our food habits, lifestyles, eating patterns, meal cycles, and portion sizes—all of which are learned. We do not eat simply for well-being and existence to obtain calories.[4] Consider only a fraction of the factors that truly influence our pattern of eating, other than those already described in this book. Food habits include the regularity of food availability and food packaging, which allow for longer availability of scarce foods. The practice of cooking expands the number and variety of foods that are edible.[5] Mealtimes (mostly culturally determined), utensils used to eat foods (norms guide utensil use for certain courses and foods), manners (self-presentation in the context of eating), and the company with whom you eat all affect your eating habits.

Lifestyle factors include income and occupation (which govern what foods are affordable), activity involved with a job, job location, and which spouse is employed. These affect meal patterns, meal preparation, and ultimately food habits.[6] What we eat is also affected by education about the nutritional value of foods,[7] ethnic identity, and religious beliefs: kosher foods for Jewish religions or abstaining from meat on Good Friday in Catholic religions, for example. Also, beliefs about health (such as vegetarianism), physiological characteristics (such as life cycle, age, or stage of development),[8] gender (usually culturally specific: for example, steak is masculine, salad is feminine), and a person's state of health all affect our eating patterns and food habits. Psychologists, dieticians, and nutritionists alike are beginning to make special considerations for these factors, which allow for culturally sensitive diet plans.[9] There is simply no such thing as an "American diet"—which is probably why Americans are prone to changing their diets so impulsively.

Based (in part) on sociocultural factors in eating, most basic models of child psychology suppose that parents and family have a primary influence over their children's diet, especially before they enter school. It reasonably follows that we should expect children to acquire diets—in the form of likes and dislikes—similar to that of their parents, since in most cases parents—either one or both—are their primary caregivers. Remarkably, though, most evidence does not support this logical progression. Paul Rozin coined the term *the family paradox* in an article demonstrating a weak association between child and parent food preferences.[10] This was true, even when comparing only mothers' preferences with their children's. Mothers not only play a larger biological role in early feeding—most early feeding experiences are via the amnion and the breast (for infants who are breast-fed)—they also traditionally have a larger role in preparing and feeding their children. It is therefore rather surprising that the preferences of mothers and their children are not well-correlated. One likely explanation may be that studies showing these weak correlations are conducted with mothers of school-aged children. Thus, it is possible that other factors (such as peer influences) could affect the child's food likes and dislikes early in life.[11]

Regardless, by now it is quite clear that each time we sit down to a meal—whether at the kitchen table, on a blanket in the park, or on the go in the car—we are experiencing a flavorful learning experience. Therefore, even without social influences, simply eating opens the door for learning and therefore shifts in dietary likes and dislikes throughout a lifespan. Still, our beliefs and attitudes, the media, moral predispositions, and even the times that we eat all can have significant impact on the diets we choose. These influences can indubitably make shifting our diets toward healthier foods more challenging; each factor will be reviewed in this chapter.

Consumer Attitudes and Media Influence

Recall from the introduction that many people diet for reasons other than a desire to be healthy. This means that many of our conceptions about foods involve how they change (body) image, not health. Americans notoriously crusade against certain nutrients, not because they are necessarily bad, but because some "expert" told them they could lose weight if they stopped consuming them. (In many cases even the experts can't say what the long-term health consequences will be.) In other words, a nutrition label is really in many cases an *image label*. This is not to imply that image is important only to adults. Children will express preferences for foods chosen by their schoolteachers,[12] fictional heroes,[13] and their peers. Indeed, recent reports indicate that brand exposure alone can significantly impact a child's taste preference—for example, children express greater preferences for foods and drinks placed in McDonald's packaging, compared to the same foods and drinks placed in unbranded packaging.[14]

Consumer attitudes toward the foods and products they buy are generally formed in two ways: central and peripheral routes.[15] These routes of attitude formation are mostly dependent on an individual's experiences and motivation. If people are motivated to understand an issue or a product (and have the ability to do so), then they are centrally motivated; otherwise, they are peripherally motivated. In terms of dietary food selection, though, very few people truly use the central route in forming attitudes about the foods they eat. For example, say you are interested in purchasing hamburger meat for a cookout. Do you care about who raised the cow, or how it was fed, nurtured, and treated (enough to stop you from making the purchase)? All of these factors would undoubtedly influence your decision to purchase and eat if you knew about them. Most cows destined for supermarkets today are fed diets of grain; but cows naturally eat grass, not grain. This diet would kill most cows, unless they receive antibiotics and hormones as part of their well-balanced diets to keep them alive. Also, most cows, while being fattened on grain, antibiotics, and hormones, are placed in close proximity to one another, where they lead very unnatural lives and would probably not live much beyond the time it takes to get them to slaughter (an estimated 5% don't make it at all). And don't be fooled: all those drugs that the farmers fed to their cows is in the meat you are feeding to your family at your cookout. [16]

With the guise of a supermarket and the prepackaging of foods, we simply don't question where our food comes from or how it was raised. We assume that the food is safe and good to eat simply because it made it to market. Our attitudes toward the foods we eat therefore are not always based on what we know; they are based mostly on what we assume. Most Americans don't even want to be informed, preferring that decisions about food safety and biotechnology be left to experts.[17] This tends to make most consumers prone to purchase foods based on peripheral attitudes toward the products they buy. In terms of food selection, we base our peripheral attitudes—and therefore which products or foods we buy—on four general factors: source credibility, labeling, emotions, and public opinion.[18]

Most people not only have favorite foods, but also favorite makers of foods. Many people will purchase name brands over the cheaper store brands, especially if they can afford to do so. Even the credibility of the endorsers or advertisers of name brands or products can determine which foods we choose. Those concerned with the health of their chickens will purchase only those labeled free-to-roam, although this is more a label than a reality—the FDA mandates that free-to-roam chickens must have access to roam; it does not mandate that they actually roam freely to be labeled as such. Tim Horton's, a popular spot for coffee in the Northeast, plays its Roll Up the Rim to Win game; McDonald's promotes its Monopoly game with a million-dollar grand prize. These promotions play on the emotions of consumers and ultimately increase profits despite having to pay the winners. The opinions of celebrities, religious leaders, scientists, daytime television personalities, and even family members can influence your decisions to select a variety of foods. Without ever checking the facts of what others say, many people will change their diets. The farther removed we are from hunting and gathering, the more *image driven* our dieting choices appear to be.

This trend (especially in Western society) does not imply that the average consumer or dieter is not intelligent; to the contrary, many peripherally influenced dieters have advanced educational backgrounds. Indeed, 83% of Americans trust the regulations set forth by the FDA, which was the second most trusted government agency behind only the Supreme Court around the turn of the twenty-first century.[19] Thus, most Americans allow the FDA to do the research for them, without ever seeking the facts themselves (i.e., their attitudes are peripherally formed). Still, while attitudes undoubtedly influence what we buy and consume, they often do not predict behavior.[20] Price and convenience are the two most common culprits behind the inconsistencies between people's attitudes and their actual consumption.[21] In fact, low prices and convenience may be the greatest reasons to eat the high-fat, high-calorie foods at fast-food restaurants. After all, you generally get more calories for your dollar when you eat there. And of course, they have convenient drive-through lanes, and they are open all night—these, along with low prices, drive people away from their attitudes about health, one convenient low-priced patty at a time. Would you like that supersized?

Moral-Social Significance

One of the strongest beliefs or attitudes an individual can have is a moral judgment. Morals are rarely violated without force and are generally considered a consequence of culture and society. They serve both to guide appropriate human behavior and to help manage the actions of man as well. Eating is no exception. Humans are notorious for establishing moral codes for what is ethical or appropriate to eat, and even include exceptions, instances in which moral codes may be violated. Consider for example the taboo associated with eating human flesh. The movie *Alive,* released in January 1993 by director Frank Marshall, describes events following the crash of a plane with 45 people on board in the Andes in October 1972. For 72 days, the victims struggled to survive, with only 16 making it. When food ran out, they survived by establishing a group norm that otherwise would have been taboo—cannibalism. When it was first suggested that they eat the flesh of the dead, the survivors dismissed it as unthinkable. Some responded that they could not do so because they would not be able to face their families if rescued. In time, though, it became their only option for survival—"from their death, we live." And when they were rescued, their families embraced them regardless. While eating human flesh is generally considered immoral, doing so to survive is acceptable (to most).

Michael Pollan writes in his book, *The Omnivore's Dilemma: A Natural History of Four Meals*, "Half the dogs in America will receive Christmas presents this year, yet few of us ever pause to consider the life of the pig—an animal easily as intelligent as a dog—that becomes the Christmas ham."[22] If asked why we don't eat the dogs and give the pigs a present, many people (especially dog lovers) would probably note that the dog is man's best friend; however, such an explanation is rooted largely in moral values. Paul Rozin noted that when Americans refuse to drink a glass of juice with a cockroach in it, they most commonly explain that the cockroach is dirty and unhealthy, a physical explanation for refusal. Yet they will reject the glass of juice even if the cockroach in the glass is dead and sterilized—in other words, it possesses no health risks to the drinker. In these cases, the reason for refusal is that "it's a cockroach!" [23]—a moral explanation.

In terms of diet, moral values generally limit which foods we can eat and even how we are judged for eating them. Whether you are one of the estimated ten million vegetarians in America, or among the greater majority of meat lovers, your moral values can (and will) affect your dietary choices. It even has been suggested that morals and values are more likely to be passed on from parent to child than preferences,[24] and this can have a significant impact on food selection. For example, researchers have demonstrated that American college students rate people who consume presumably healthier diets (such as salads, fruits, whole-wheat breads, etc.) as more moral and considerate (as opposed to virtuous and inconsiderate).[25] On the other hand, those consuming less-healthy diets (such as steaks, hamburgers, French fries, etc.) were rated as much less moral and considerate. Thus, even the foods that we consider morally appropriate to consume are subject to moral judgments (as are the people who eat them).

Ultimately, our moral judgments about the foods we eat (and don't eat) will affect what we choose to include in our diets. At some level, it is likely that we are aware of this. Social psychologists have often noted that we behave differently in groups than we do alone, partly because we assume that those in the group are judging our behavior. For example, we tend to eat more food when others are eating more food; we tend to eat healthier foods when others are making healthier choices; we tend to take smaller portions of foods when others are doing the same. Concerns for moral judgments regarding eating, health, and body image undoubtedly influence how we behave among a group, especially among peers with whom we are not familiar.

Food Selection and Time of Day

How we select which foods to eat (and how much of it to eat) is dependent on a variety of factors: preferences, aversions, feelings of hunger and satiety, routes of attitude formation, moral significance, and social, cultural, economic, and biological factors (to name a few). These interact to affect which foods and how much food we choose to consume. More than this, we don't simply select *which* foods to consume; we select *when* to consume them. Certain foods have appropriate times to be eaten.

Americans consider eggs, bacon, pancakes, and cereals to be appropriate breakfast foods; cold-cut sandwiches, soups, and "leftovers" for lunch; and hot, prepared foods (such as pastas or stir fry) with multiple courses (often including salads and desserts) for dinner. Therefore, the acceptability of foods is determined largely by the context or timing of our appetites.[26] Anecdotal evidence from my research indicates that many people assume others share their expectations about the appropriateness of foods for eating at certain times. For example, I used a variety of foods in a study that found people who consume snack foods eat more afterward (see chapter 3). For the study, I tried to pick foods that some people thought of as snack foods and other people considered to be meal foods. The foods used in the study included pasta salad, potato salad, jelly sandwiches, cheese sandwiches, turkey, roast beef, honey-roasted ham, and bologna (either rolled up and held with a toothpick or served as a thick slice). In discussions with my esteemed colleagues, it became obvious that our opinions were polarized. Each person was convinced that he or she could divide these selections into categories of meal foods and snack foods, and that all of the subjects in my study would see things the same way. But they didn't. When asked in a preliminary questionnaire how they perceived these foods, some participants responded that foods such as pasta salad, potato salad, and jelly sandwiches were snack foods, while others indicated that these same foods were meal foods. As it turns out, how we think of food varies from one individual to another and since how we think of food significantly affects our dieting choices (and how much we consume), this reinforces the notion that one diet simply cannot fit all.

Still, we have established norms for which foods go together and what order foods should be eaten within a meal. These sociocultural norms can affect food selection and acceptability. For example, some people put ketchup on their eggs, while others wouldn't think of combining those foods; chocolate goes with milk, but not with cola; pizza goes with chicken wings, French fries, chicken strips, celery, carrots, and dips, but most would not combine these foods with other vegetables such as corn and mashed potatoes (which many people like, especially with added high-fat butter). Also, meals (especially dinners) are often served in courses. If your mom was anything like mine, there was absolutely no dessert before dinner (or any other meal) because "you'll spoil your appetite!" Of course, by dessert I do not mean a salad, but a high-calorie cookie, some crackers, or a slice of cake. However, it should be evident that this tradition is one that many families might want to reconsider (see the discussion on the dessert effect in chapter 8).

We eat what we like, and we like different foods and nutrients at different times of the day before or after some foods and together with certain other foods. Each of us is essentially a *psychological dieter*, negotiating the omnivore's dilemma to consume healthier diets through a psychology of eating that is seemingly impervious to the calories we actually consume.

Society and Culture: A Clinical Application

The psychological dieter is a person who "hunts" for food in supermarkets and at the drive-through. He or she is the dieter whose issues do not concern how to obtain food, but instead how to select among the foods available. For the psychological dieter, the challenge is not whether there is food to eat, but whether he or she will eat healthy foods. We live in a world that makes food readily available, easy to access, and more affordable than ever, and that presumably takes the guesswork out of whether the foods we consume are safe (at least in developed countries). With all this has come, ironically, a surge in disease and deaths directly or indirectly related to the foods we eat. This has serious clinical implications for healthcare. Although solutions have been proposed in the United States, nothing seems to be working—at least on a large scale with long-term success—and the failure to fully appreciate sociocultural and economic factors may be at least partly to blame.

Let's consider a clinical example with black-American minorities, who constitute a significant proportion of the American population. Among members of this group the unemployment rate is more than double that of white Americans. On average, they earn less income and obtain less education than white Americans, and nearly one-third live below the poverty line. The life expectancy for black males is shorter than for any other group in the United States. Many depend on subsidies to live, including the Women, Infants, and Children program (WIC), food stamps, school breakfast and lunch programs, and emergency food programs.[27] Being on such programs often results in stigmatization, especially when people use food stamps as currency to purchase basic food necessities at supermarkets.

Consider just a few of the challenges facing a significant percentage of the members of this group. Working habits alter eating patterns, researchers find, and many black-Americans are blue-collar workers, work inflexible hours, and tend to be disrupted by irregular meal schedules—family members eat when convenient, and many consume fast-food diets. These factors tend to be associated more with socioeconomic status (which is primarily determined by income level) than simply with race,[28] but this doesn't make the problem go away. In fact, while lower socioeconomic status is associated with a greater tendency for dieting and bingeing among women,[29] it is also associated with greater rates of obesity in both men and women—and these factors have serious implications for minority health in America today.

Black American women are the least likely to seek prenatal care or to breast-feed their children,[30] which results in the highest percentage of preterm births, low-birth weight infants, and rate of infant deaths in the United States. In traditional black American culture—especially in the Southern states—food is a catalyst for social interaction. Health concerns include nutritional deficiencies (especially in the elderly[31]) caused by insufficient food intake, not a poor diet per se. One study found that poor urban black Americans consume higher nutrient density diets (including diets high in fat) than white Americans of similar socioeconomic status.[32] Black American diets are also associated with insufficient consumption of vitamins, fruits, vegetables, and fiber products,[33] all of which are likely attributable to a range of social and cultural factors limiting the variety and timeliness of their diets.

In addition, black Americans (men and women) have the highest incidence of cancer and deaths resulting from cancer in the United States. Their rate of deaths resulting from cancer is estimated to be more than twice that of all other minorities combined. Black Americans also have the highest death rates (by far) resulting from diabetes, heart disease, and strokes of any ethnicity or race in the United States. Moreover, the rates of obesity among black Americans are higher than any other race in the country. As of 2005, it was estimated that 68% of this minority group are clinically overweight or obese; about 9% above the national average. One cultural caveat in regard to the obesity statistics—one that is well-documented—is that black American men have more permissive attitudes regarding obesity than do other races.[34] Black men are more likely to prefer women with "a little meat on their bones." Still, statistics indicate that this minority group is especially prone to disease and death linked either directly or indirectly to what they eat. Improving healthcare—at the patient and fiscal level—requires that we address these culturally specific health facts to create real solutions.[35]

The clinical implications for this minority group are overwhelming to consider. This group generally has inadequate access to healthcare, low incomes, and high unemployment rates that contribute to the healthcare problem. Yet while these are the issues facing one-third of all black Americans, the majority of dieting strategies aimed at improving long-term health requires involved medical interventions (both surgical and behavioral) that would require time, money, and health insurance—all of which are generally difficult to come by for this minority group. While culturally based approaches can allow for diets that are easier to maintain, provide greater attention to the individual, and eventually reduce health risks,[36] these strategies must be relatively simple, short-term, and cost-effective to be successful on a large scale. Considering minorities are expected to account for over half of the American population two decades from now, ignoring strategies that address their sociocultural and economic needs (as they pertain to health and diet) will only increase the problems associated with a healthcare system that is barely capable of managing American health today.

The Psychological Dieter: A Final Thought

The psychological principles discussed in this book undoubtedly have the potential to address the three main sociocultural and economic factors that limit large-scale dieting success—strategies that are *simple, short-term,* and *cost-effective*. Strategies for increasing fullness and shifting liking to lower calorie, healthier food options are indeed simple and cost-effective: any individual could apply these strategies—all they have to do is buy the food. Just as important, these strategies are short-term, taking only a few days or weeks in most cases to cause permanent shifts in the person's diet. They require only that healthy, low-calorie foods be introduced to a person's pleasurable diet. In short, research in psychology shows us that shifting human diet long-term requires that we adapt to how we learn about fullness and liking—not by counting calories.

Still, eating healthy is not so simple for most dieters. When you consider all of the factors that affect eating, it is no wonder so many people jump from one diet to another, swearing by a diet until it fails the person—and most diets eventually will. Whether we feel hungry or full depends at least as much on what we learn about foods as it does on innate biology. This is also true with liking and disliking—most likes and dislikes are learned, and there is no evidence that we ever stop learning. While our biology is such that it works hard to maintain us on a diet that works—meaning one that keeps us alive—the diet it keeps us on is not always going to be the healthiest diet. In most cases, our diets are probably unhealthy for long-term dieting, thanks in large part to our innate biology. Of course, we live much longer now, making our dieting choices that much more important for long-term health—it was only 100 years ago that life expectancy for humans was about forty years of age (less than half what it is today). We are living in a new world with an evolutionarily outdated body that is not designed for our *feast and feast some more* existence. Solutions for dieting success must address this, lest we continue this failed dieting cycle until the day we choose to embrace our starring role as *the psychological dieter*.

Notes

1. Birch, L. L., Zimmerman, S., & Hind, H. (1980). The influence of social-affective context on preschool children's food preferences. *Child Development, 51*, 856-861.
2. Birch, L. L., Birch, D., Marlin, D., & Kramer, L. (1982). Effects of instrumental eating on children's food preferences. *Appetite, 3*, 125-134.
3. Batsell, W. R., Jr., Brown, A. S., Ansfield, M. E., & Paschall, G. Y. (2002). "You will eat all of that!'": A retrospective analysis of forced consumption episodes. *Appetite, 38*, 211-219.
4. Lowenberg, M. E. (1970). Socio-cultural basis of food habits. *Food Technology, 24*, 27-32.
5. Fernandez-Armesto, F. (2002). *Near a thousand tables: A history of food*. New York: Free Press.
6. Pelto, G. H. (1981). Anthropological contributions to nutrition education research. *Journal of Nutrition Education, 13* (supplement), S2-S8.
7. Kempson K., Keenan, D. P., Sadani, P. S., & Adler, A. (2003). Maintaining food sufficiency: Coping strategies identified by limited-resource individuals versus nutrition educations. *Journal of Nutrition Education & Behavior, 35* (4), 179-188.
8. Rozin, P. N., & Schulkin, J. (1990). Food selection. In Stricker, E. M. (Ed). *Neurobiology of Food and Fluid Intake: Handbook of Behavioral Neurobiology, vol. 10* (pp. 297-328), New York: Plenum Press.

9. Axelson, M. L. (1986). The impact of culture on food-related behavior. *Annual Review of Nutrition, 6*, 345-363.
10. Rozin, P. (1991). Family resemblance in food and other domains: The family paradox and the role of family congruence. *Appetite, 16*, 93-102.
11. Birch, L. L. (1980). Effect of peer model's food choices and eating behaviors on pre-schoolers' food preferences. *Child Development, 51*, 489-496.
12. Birch, L. L., Zimmerman, S. I., & Hind, H. (1980). The influence of social-affective context on the formation of children's food preferences. *Child Development, 51*, 856-861.
13. Marinho, H. (1942). Social influence in the formation of enduring preferences. *Journal of Abnormal and Social Psychology, 37*, 448-468.
14. Robinson, T. N., Borzekowski, D. L. G., Matheson, D. M., & Kraemer, H. C. (2007). Effects of fast food branding on young children's taste preferences. *Arch. Pediatr. Adolesc. Med.*, 161 (8), 792-797.
15. Petty, R. E., & Cacioppo, J. T. (1981). *Attitudes and persuasion: Classic and contemporary approaches*. Dubuque, IA: Brown.
16. For a compelling discussion read Pollan, M. (2006). The omnivore's dilemma: A natural history of four meals. New York: Penguin Press.
17. Optima Consultants. (1994). *Understanding the consumer interest in the new biotechnology industry* (report prepared for the Office of Consumer Affairs, Ottawa). Ottawa, Canada: Industry Canada.
18. Wansink, B., & Kim, J. (2001). The marketing battle over genetically modified foods: False assumptions about consumer behavior. *American Behavioral Scientist*, 44 (8), 1405-1417.
19. Hadfield, G., Howse, R., & Trebilcock, M. J. (1998). Information-based principles biotechnology is influenced not only by their perceptions about the magnitude of the for rethinking consumer protection policy. *Journal of Consumer Policy, 21*, 131-169.
20. Heijs, W. J. M., & Midden, C. .J. H. (1995). *Biotechnology: Attitudes and Influencing Factors, Third Survey*. Eindhoven, The Netherlands: Eindhoven University of Technology.
21. Wansink, B., & Ray, M. L. (1992). Estimating an advertisement's impact on one's consumption of a brand. *Journal of Advertising Research, 26* (4), 9-16.
22. Pollan, M. (2006). *The Omnivore's Dilemma: A Natural History of Four Meals* (citation on pp. 306). New York: Penguin Press.
23. Rozin, P. (1996). Sociocultural influences on human food selection. In E. D. Capaldi, *Why We Eat What We Eat: The Psychology of Eating* (pp. 233-263). Washington, D.C.: American Psychological Association.
24. Cavalli-Sforza, L. L., Feldman, M. W., Chen, K. H., & Dornbusch, S. M. (1982). Theory and observation in cultural transmission. *Science, 218*, 19-27.
25. Stein, R. I., & Nemeroff, C. J. (1995). Moral overtones of food: Judgments of others based on what they eat. *Personality and Social Psychology Bulletin, 21*, 480-490.
26. Rozin, P., & Tuorila, H. (1993). Simultaneous and temporal contextual influences on food choice. *Food Quality and Preference, 4*, 11-20.
27. Lee, B. J., Mackey-Bilaver, L., & George, R. M. (2003). The patterns of Food Stamp and WIC participation under welfare reform. *Children & Youth Services Review, 25* (8), 589-610.

28. Gerber, A. M., James, S. A., Ammerman, A. S., Keenan, N. L., & Brussel, J. A. (1991). Socioeconomic status and electrolyte intake in Black adults: The Pitt County study. *American Journal of Public Health*, 81 (12), 1608-1612.

29. Drewnowski, A., Kurth, C. L., & Krahn, D. D. (1994). Body weight and dieting in adolescence: Impact of socioeconomic status. *International Journal of Eating Disorders*, 16 (1), 61-65.

30. Kittler, P. G., & Sucher, K. (1995). *Food and Culture in America*. St. Paul, MN: West Publishing Company.

31. Sharkey, J. R., & Schoenberg, N. E. (2002). Variations in Nutritional Risk Among Black and White Women Who Receive Home-Delivered Meals. *Journal of Women & Aging*, 14 (3-4), 99-119.

32. Emmons, L. (1986). Food procurement and the nutritional adequacy of diets in low-income families. *Journal of the American Dietetic Association, 86*, 1684-1693.

33. Lokken, S. L., Byrd, S., & Hope, K. J. (2002). Assessing nutrition risk and sociodemographic characteristics of low-income older adults living in Mississippi. *Journal of Nutrition for the Elderly*, 21 (4), 21-37.

34. Kumanyika, S. (1987). Obesity in black women. *Epidemiologic Reviews, 9*, 31-50.

35. Unless otherwise noted, statistics and data reported for African-Americans were taken from the http://statehealthfacts.org website.

36. Xie, B., Gilliland, F. D., Li, Y., & Rockett, H. R. (2003). Effects of ethnicity, family income, and education on dietary intake among adolescents. *Preventive Medicine*, 36 (1), 30-40.

About the Author

Born in Buffalo, New York, Gregory J. Privitera served four honorable years in the United States Marine Corps before entering college and two additional years with the New York Army National Guard while attending college. He received multiple academic degrees in psychology leading to a doctoral degree (Ph.D.) from The State University of New York at Buffalo. Today, Gregory is an Assistant Professor at Glendale Community College in Glendale, AZ, and a Faculty Associate at Arizona State University in Tempe, AZ, where he teaches on topics in psychology and oversees laboratory research projects. His research and career is focused on understanding how principles in psychology can be used to improve health and well-being, and his work was recently recognized with the publication of his biography in the prestigious *Who's Who of Emerging Leaders* in 2007.

www.ingramcontent.com/pod-product-compliance
Lightning Source LLC
Chambersburg PA
CBHW020357270326
41926CB00007B/483

9 780761 839668